SNATCHED TO PERFECTION

My Journey with Diastasis Recti & the Truth about Cosmetic Surgery

Trell Taylor

Snatched to Perfection:
My Journey with Diastasis Recti
& the Truth about Cosmetic Surgery

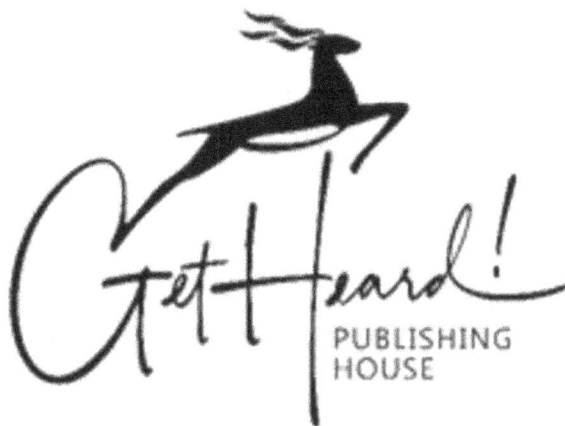

PUBLISHING HOUSE

Paperback: 978-1-964111-29-2
Hardcover: 978-1-964111-30-8

Dedication

To my dear children, Patrick and Jeremiah, you are my heartbeats, my world, my inspiration, and the reasons I strive to provide for you.

Remember that everything in life is a learning lesson, a test, and ultimately a testimony. "Snatched to Perfection" exemplifies how motherhood has taught me so much about myself, both emotionally and physically. It has pushed me to dig deep, work hard, and gain a better understanding of myself and what it means to be a mother. Because of the lessons I've learned and the challenges I've faced, I now have a testimony to share with others to guide them on their journey toward perfection.

Thank you for equipping, believing in, and inspiring me. I love you both! -Mom

Table of Contents

Preface

The increasing focus on body image through social media, television, books, and music has mounted even more pressure for women to have a particular look. Each year brings new terminology describing the perfect look, and in the urban community, one term that represents the perfect body, a small waist with rounded hips and buttocks, is "snatched." I exercised. I hired a trainer. I exercise more, and while I saw some changes, I still couldn't achieve the snatched version I hoped for. Then, I discovered that I suffered from an actual medical condition, diastasis recti. Though you may be unfamiliar with this term, we are all familiar with the desire to feel confident and whole.

Although I had given birth to two beautiful baby boys and was proud to be their mother, I did not feel confident and whole afterward. My body was different, and as much as I tried to embrace that difference, clothes that didn't fit appropriately remained a constant reminder of what I could not achieve on my own. The only fix was cosmetic surgery. The thought of cosmetic surgery absolutely scared me because of all the horror stories you hear. Yet, in the process of my journey, I learned that this medical condition was common among mothers, and I questioned how many were dealing with this hidden monster. My focus shifted from simply wanting to share my journey toward the perfect body to educating others about what it took to solve it, but as my writing journey unfolded, some other profound truths emerged, ones that formed in the early part of my childhood.

As early as grade school, societal expectations and sometimes our failed attempts at what we think we should look like or be have left all of us facing the challenge of what is considered perfection. I remember the first time I was aware of my looks and the disappointment I felt. It was the moment that shaped my understanding of image. As you read my story, you may see pieces of your journey reflected here. If you do, don't hesitate to share your stories with me. Your experiences can help others going through similar struggles. Also, as you read, I want you to take away a few key points. First, choose confidence by embracing who you are, no matter what you face. Second, you will need to make some decisions that others may not agree with or have negative opinions about. Still, you have to decide what is best for your situation. Third, happiness is real. Self-love is real. You need both. Finally, inspire someone else. Your story can do for them what this story will do for you.

-Trell Taylor

Acknowledgements

No such thing as a solo journey exists, especially one like this. First and foremost, I want to thank God for giving me the strength to endure every sleepless night, every moment of doubt, and every ache, itch, and tear. I would not have made it through the first night without my faith in God and the power of prayer.

To my family, who saw me at my lowest and most vulnerable, thank you for your patience, support, and understanding when I struggled to even sit up on my own.

To my friends who checked on me, brought food, listened to my complaints, and reminded me that I wasn't alone; your love lifted me.

To my medical team, from the surgeon to the nurses and everyone who answered my panicked, late-night questions, thank you for your care, compassion, and for being honest and patient with me through it all.

To everyone who has gone through this journey before me and to those still navigating it, you have inspired me. Your vulnerability, transparency, and strength matter more than you know.

Finally, to each person reading this book, thank you for your time, openness, and willingness to look deeper than just the "before and after." You are the reason I wrote this.

This book is for us, those who choose to rewrite our narratives, own our choices, embrace our scars, and celebrate our transformations. We understand that perfection is not the absence of flaws; it is about healing and having the confidence to define beauty on our own terms. It is about the bold decision to reclaim our bodies in our own way!

With love,
Trell Taylor

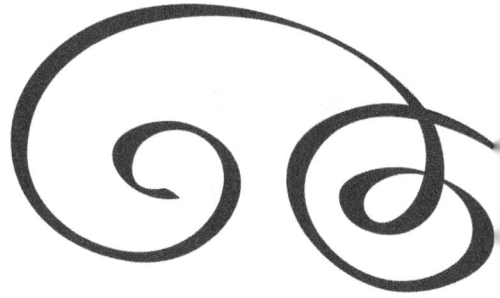

Introduction
Another Typical Day

It was another typical day for me. Clothes lay strewn across the bed as I tried to figure out what would work best. Frustration lay bare. What was I going to wear? As I looked in the mirror, I criticized every inch of my body, some areas more than others. My family and friends often complimented me on how beautiful I was, but what they saw, I could not. And what they could not see when they looked at me was the smoothing waist trainers plus the tummy control pants. I know we are our own worst critics, and it is our personal critiques that matter and drive our thoughts, not necessarily what others think. Reality is that everyone will have their opinions about how you look, even if positive. Yet for me, it all becomes irrelevant as I peel off the layers of tummy control and other shapewear, revealing the real me when I turn my hips and see the sides of my body or the extra skin on my back.

We're familiar with the phrase, If you're unhappy with your appearance when looking in the mirror, do something about it. It's easier said than done, right? For some, dieting, working out, other lifestyle changes, and even good genetics easily help them shed the pounds in the areas that haunt them. I was not in this group, but among the other group of people, the ones who had tried everything. Because of possible interference due to genetics or a medical condition, such as in my situation with diastasis recti, we cannot do it. For well over ten years, I struggled, asking myself how I was supposed to get snatched to perfection, and I didn't even know what I was working with. Even when I conducted a personal poll, only about ten percent of women knew about diastasis recti and how it affected their ability to lose weight and achieve their snatched perfection.

When I look back at those moments, I think about the number of times I was embarrassed by my looks or questioned whether I would look good enough by my husband's side. However, he had always been highly supportive of me and never failed to tell me how beautiful I looked. Still, I cannot help but think about all the other moms who are experiencing what I experienced: clothes strewn across the bed, questioning themselves in the mirror, wondering why they could not achieve the snatched perfection they sought. In my journey, I discovered that it is an issue of duality: the gap between what the mind perceives and the actual physical challenge you may face. So my quest for **snatched to perfection** began.

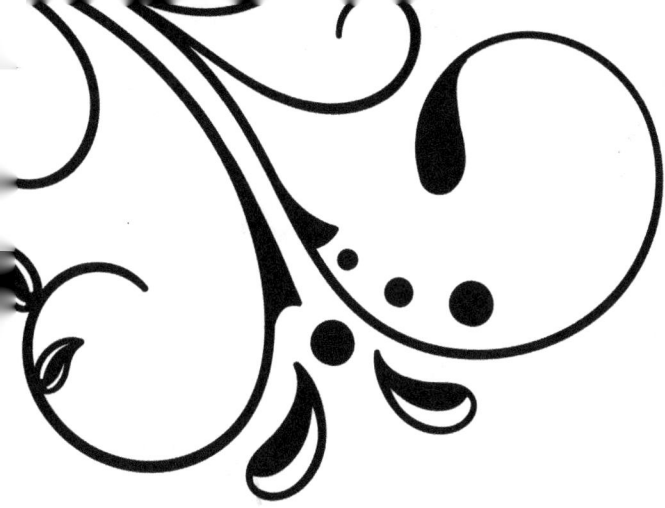

"The noise was deafening, intense. I couldn't hear myself think. I attempted to run away quickly, but they ran even faster, as if chasing me down like a wolf on the trail of its prey."

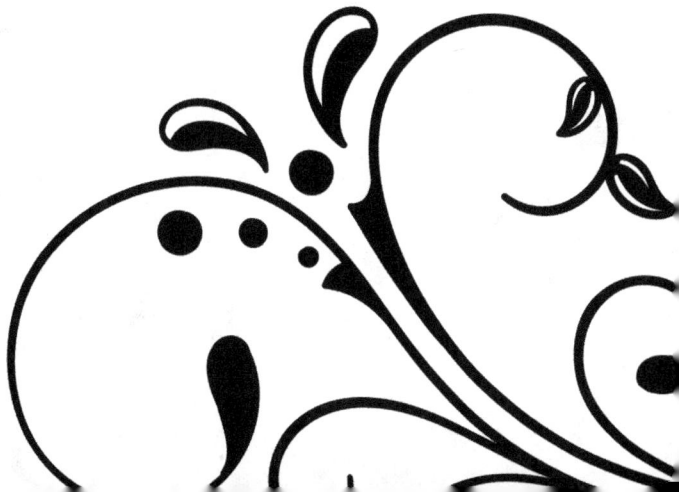

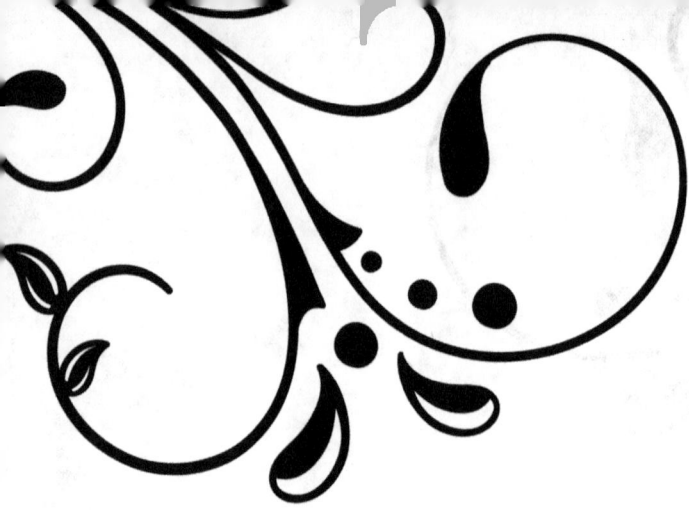

"My face wet with a mixture of salty tears and sweat beaming down my cheeks, I felt like my feet were a ton of bricks. I wanted to run but couldn't."

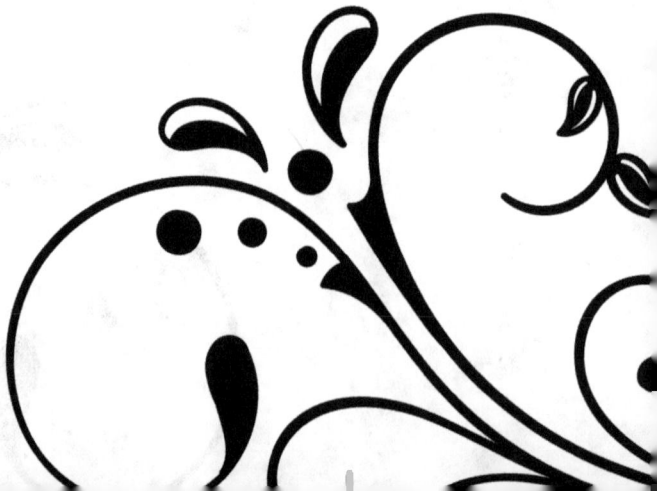

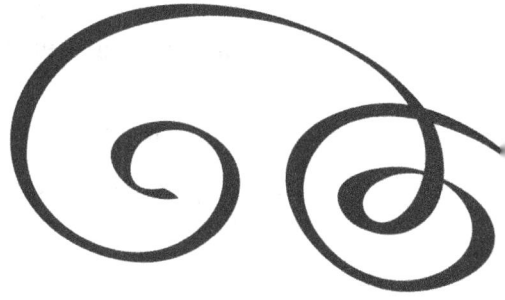

Chapter 1
Image Is Everything
Splinter the Rat

Sixth grade is when the torture began for me. That is when I realized that the image actually mattered to people. Before that, I had never thought about what I looked like until that dreaded day. That's when the teasing started.

My friends and I were on the playground, playing kickball like kids do at recess. Suddenly, I heard a voice from across the playground; it was Michael. I never liked him because I thought he was rude and arrogant. At first, I ignored him, assuming he was playing with his friends, just as I was. But his voice got louder and closer.

I quickly turned around, only to find Michael standing right behind me. He wasn't alone; his friend Ezekiel was next to him, grinning like a Cheshire cat. Fear washed over me because I had no clue why they were behind me, smiling in such a mischievous way. My heart raced, and my hands began to sweat. I felt a lump in my throat the size of a golf ball as I swallowed in fear. I was terrified. Michael and Ezekiel were notorious for terrorizing other sixth graders, and today, it seemed, I was their chosen victim.

He Called Me a Rat!

Then it began, those words that I will never forget! Michael and Ezekiel started singing, "Splinter, Splinter, Splinter; Trell is a Splinter." I was so confused. My hands were sweating, and my face felt just as damp. Sweat dripped down my back, as well as down my face and onto my mouth, the saltiness settling across my tongue. *Why are they calling me Splinter?* I wondered. I turned to walk away, but they and their friends followed closely behind me, getting closer with each line of the song. Soon, everyone was singing along with them. The noise was deafening, intense. I couldn't hear myself think. I attempted to run away quickly, but they ran even faster, as if chasing me down like a wolf on the trail of its prey.

Abruptly, I stopped and screamed, "Why are you calling me Splinter? That's not my name!"

Michael replied, "It is your name now, Splinter, because you're like the rat from *Teenage Mutant Ninja Turtles*." Everyone, including Ezekiel, erupted in laughter, the sound echoing around the playground as if it were bouncing off the walls of a glass cage. I was trapped with no way to escape. Yet, confusion continued to grip me as my thoughts swirled. Splinter? I didn't even like the show *Teenage Mutant Ninja Turtles*.

Sensing my confusion, Michael obliged me with an explanation by placing his thumb underneath his two top middle teeth and said, "Buckteeth Splinter, buckteeth Splinter, Trell is a buckteeth Splinter!" Then it dawned on me. *Is that why everyone called my father "Rat," and some people even call him "Super Rat"? Why would he be okay with that?* I immediately began to get upset with my father. After all, I inherited my tooth deformities from him, and so did my brother and sister. *Why didn't he fix his teeth so that we wouldn't have bad teeth? Why would he be okay with being teased? Now, I was being teased because he didn't fix his teeth before I was born. Had he fixed his teeth, I would not have had bad teeth,* I thought to myself.

I immediately burst into tears hearing this because even if my father was okay with being called "Rat," I hated being called that. My face wet with a mixture of salty tears and sweat beaming down my cheeks, I felt like my feet were a ton of bricks. I wanted to run but couldn't. I stood in the center of the crowd, barely able to open my eyes, as the laughter and taunting continued. I fell to my knees, wondering where the teachers were. *Where were my friends who were playing with me earlier? Were they laughing and singing too?* It felt like I was trapped in a dream, unable to wake up. I lay on the ground for what felt like hours until the bell rang. When it did, the crowd dispersed as if nothing had happened. I was finally free, or so I thought. The taunting didn't end there; almost every day after that, I would hear the Splinter song. I never spoke up; I only endured it each time. Eventually, I grew tired of the teasing and reached a breaking point.

The Bus Ride Home

My breaking point happened on a Friday afternoon during the bus ride home from school. Andrew teased, "Splinter, Splinter, Splinter. Trell is a buckteeth Splinter." Perhaps I had had a long day, or maybe I had just taken one too many jokes.

Whatever it was, it was long overdue. As I sat in my seat on the bus, Andrew not only sang the "Splinter song," but he was beating on the back of my seat. He was a drummer at his church and was now treating my seat as though it were his drums while he sang the song.

I could feel myself becoming angrier. I turned around and yelled, "Stop, Andrew!" Of course, he would not stop, and instead, got louder with the song and beat more intensely on the back of my seat. He laughed hysterically as he looked at the anger in my face. I clenched my hands into a tight fist. All I could think of was shutting him up. I started to stand, but sat back down, which made him get louder. Instinctively, I turned completely around and swung my clenched fist right into his jaw, knocking him out of his seat. I was fuming at that point and only saw red. *Did I really hit him?* I thought to myself. I was so proud of myself that I jumped on top of him, continuously swinging with all of my strength, hitting him in the face over and over again until I was out of breath. The bus driver slammed on the brakes, and we went flying down the aisle of the bus. I was still on top of him, fighting. The bus driver came and pulled me off of him and separated us, yelling at me. She didn't bother to ask who started it or what happened, and honestly, I really didn't care. I was just happy that I shut him up. Now I was the one grinning like a Cheshire cat as I looked at the large cartoon knots all over his swollen face.

I taunted him, saying, "You got beat up by a girl Splinter; you got beat up by a girl Splinter!" Some people may have seen me as Splinter with buckteeth, but in that moment, I saw Andrew as the cartoon knot head. Sixth grade was when I first learned that image was everything.

Fitting In

Once I went to middle school, the name-calling was not as nasty as it was in sixth grade, although it still occurred. I tried to be more outgoing so that my classmates could see me as a person, not "Splinter the Buckteeth Rat." Despite my attempts, that name followed me around. It was not until I moved away to a different school district that I finally had an opportunity to obtain a new image.

When I started high school, I was still the same skinny girl from Columbus, MS, weighing barely ninety pounds. Although I was not happy with my appearance, I considered myself a decent-looking person with chocolate skin, straight black hair, and dark brown, dreamy eyes. People often told me I was cute, and I held onto that compliment after enduring years of being called "Splinter." However, being cute just wasn't enough for me. I wanted to be part of the popular crowd, the girls everyone adored. But how could a skinny, buck-toothed girl like me become popular? I didn't know the answer, but I was determined to find out.

I watched videos and television shows that focused on having the perfect body and image. I realized that everything I saw featured outgoing girls with beautiful faces, long curly hair, tight-fitting clothes, big earrings, red lipstick, and colorful makeup. How could I ever compare to that? I was a quiet and shy kid with shoulder-length straight hair, an average face with pimples, regular-fitting clothes, small gold dot earrings, and lip gloss, because my mother would never allow me to wear makeup or lipstick at my age. I thought there was no chance I would ever become popular like the girls on television. This realization saddened me, and I felt that I would forever be known as "Splinter the Buckteeth Rat." Yet, it dawned on me: I was in a completely different school! They knew me as Trell, not Splinter. Hmmm, maybe I had a chance at a normal high school life after all. However, I still longed for popularity, which seemed so unreachable to me. So, I went the route most teenagers try first, fitting in.

The more I tried to fit in, the more I felt like a failure. I was a new girl at a new school, trying desperately to get away from the constant torture that I felt since sixth grade. Even though I was at a new school, my mind was stuck on their words, "Trell, the Bucktooth Splinter," and I couldn't shake it. Instead of fitting in, my days became lonelier. Academically, I excelled. Socially, sometimes, I wish I could disappear. My social skills were horrible. Every night, I thought hard about how to fit in, and every morning, I dreaded going to school because I had no answers. Then, one day, my Spanish teacher introduced me to the Spanish club because of my excellent Spanish grades. That day became the pivotal moment that changed my life.

The Plan

Once I joined the Spanish club, I thought that this was what I needed to do to become more popular, but what other clubs could I join? My mind was always racing a "mile a minute," as my mother would say. She was always concerned about my silence, but she always told me that I could talk to her about anything. The problem is that I never told her or anyone about how I felt or how I was teased. I dealt with it internally, as I did many other things in my life, which I later discovered was not the best approach. However, I was determined to figure it out on my own and see how I could fix this problem. I started joining every club or organization that I could think of, regardless of their activities or potential benefits. I know. I know. It was not a smart idea, but I did not care. I absolutely had to become popular like the girls on television.

I joined the modeling squad, Archonettes of Zeta Phi Beta Sorority, Incorporated (which actually became a wise decision for my college plans), and the basketball cheerleading team. You see, I wasn't at any school; I went to New Hope High School, where image was everything; well, at least, I thought so. Once I joined various organizations and clubs, I knew one of them would help me achieve my goal of becoming more popular. That was my mission in life, and nothing else mattered. Every organization was pretty easy to join, except the basketball cheerleading team. I was not going to let that stop me, though.

Cheerleaders are supposed to be loud and outgoing, expected to have specific skills, but I didn't care. For this quiet and shy girl, image was the focus. Knowing I couldn't tumble at all, I stuck to basketball cheerleading; no tumbling for us on a basketball court compared to tumbling on a football field as a football cheerleader. It was a win-win for me. That is, if I made the team. The only experience that I had as a cheerleader was from the ages of seven to nine, where my friends and I had cheering wars with the neighborhood kids who thought they were better and cuter than us. Even then, at that age, this idea of image was everything raised its ugly head. I just wasn't as aware of it at that age. Perhaps those cheering wars helped because I made the team.

Confidence Booster

Not knowing what I was getting myself into, I was super excited because all I could see was that I would now be popular. As soon as I got off the bus, I raced home to tell my mother. I raced as though I were in a marathon. I saw people watching and probably wondering what was wrong and why I was running so fast. I didn't care because I had to share the news with my mother.

I burst into the front door, knocking over everything that was in my way. I ran into the living room, through the kitchen, and finally into her room, where I found her. I was so tired; I could barely speak to share the news. I stuttered over my words, and she immediately began to worry, asking what was wrong and what had happened. I was so out of breath from running that my words made no sense as they were coming out of my mouth. She grabbed some water for me, which I gulped down so fast that I choked on it. Her eyes were so big, and I could see the fear in them because she didn't know what was wrong.

Finally, I calmed myself down enough to scream the words, "I made the basketball cheerleading team!" I expected her to share my excitement, my joy. She was happy but seemed worried.

"Baby, how are you going to be a cheerleader with you being so quiet and shy?" I had no clue, but one thing that I did know was that I was going to be popular, and that's all that mattered.

The cute little cheerleader uniforms boosted my confidence and image. During the game season, I gradually overcame some of my shyness. However, it wasn't until I became a member of the best sorority in college, Zeta Phi Beta Sorority, Incorporated, that I was more sociable and less shy, despite being an Archonette in high school. Nevertheless, I couldn't wait for game days to wear my uniform. I interacted more with the basketball players because we did treat bags for them and spirit signs for game days. I dated one of the basketball players, Richard. I absolutely loved everything about being a cheerleader because my mission was finally a success. I had more friends and popularity, which was all I ever dreamed of. Image was important, but when my senior year rolled around, the idea that image was everything really took hold.

I remained on the cheer squad through my senior year in high school. That year, our cheerleader uniforms were white, sparkly, and wait for it... had a slit on the thigh! You could not tell me anything because, again, image was everything. I had put on a little weight, now weighing a hundred pounds, and fit perfectly into my new uniform! In the past, I hated looking in the mirror because my body wasn't as full as some of my peers'. Now at one hundred pounds and filling out my uniform, I loved looking in the mirror. The braces were gone, and I was slowly beginning to love what I saw. I looked in the mirror every chance that I got, eyeing my body in my cheerleader suit, sticking my thigh out of the slit, and I had even grown breasts. Yes! And so it began, the obsession with remaining *snatched to perfection*.

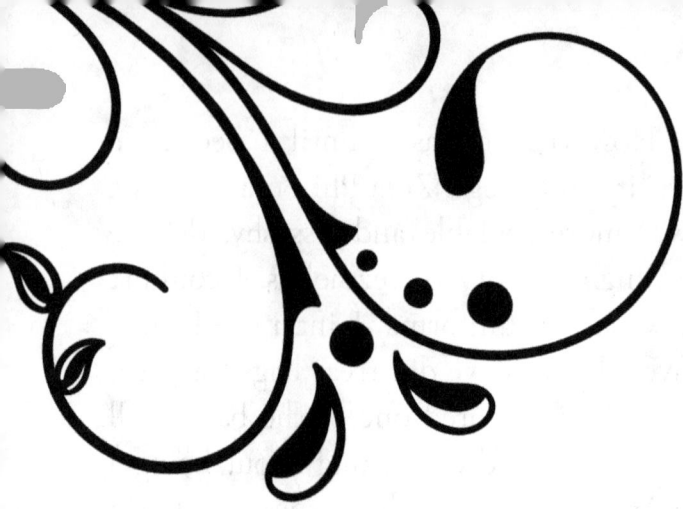

"As I sat on the toilet seat, sweating, I started sniffing and crying. I tried to speak, but I couldn't."

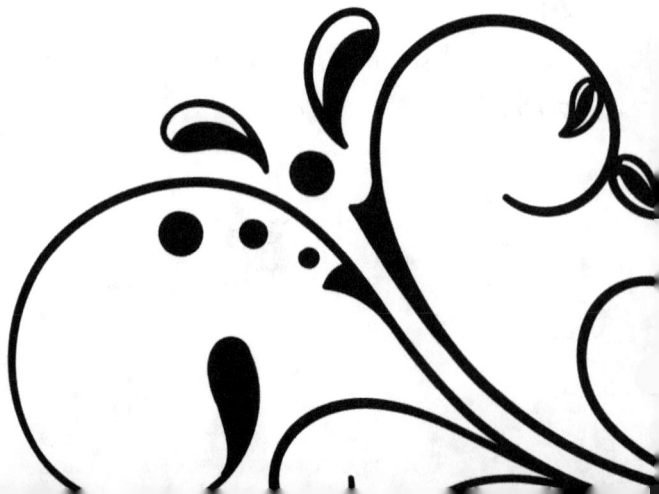

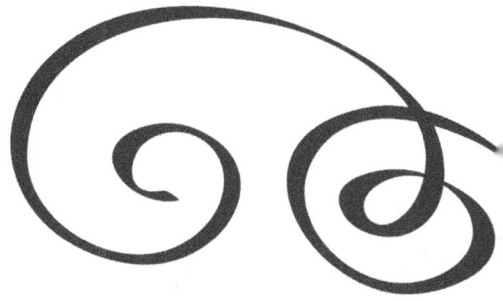

Chapter 2
The Unplanned Mommy Makeover
The Doughnut Belly

Fast forward twenty-five years, and I looked in the mirror and could only see a nightmare. Long gone was the perfectly slim one-hundred-pound girl, who loved to stick her thigh through the cheer uniform slit. Though everyone told me I was overreacting or exaggerating about my body because nothing was wrong, I could not see myself differently. To me, I looked like an overweight cartoon character with a doughnut-shaped belly.

In high school, I knew exactly what I wanted my future to look like and wrote it down in my senior year memory book. I wanted to attend Mississippi State University (MSU), relocate to Memphis, Tennessee, secure a job in accounting, work at International Paper, and have my first child by the time I was twenty-five. As a thirty-year-old mother, I looked back at my memory book and realized that I had accomplished every single one of my dreams. I attended MSU, moved to Memphis, and started working at International Paper as a Financial

Analyst/Accountant. And wait for it, I was pregnant at twenty-five years old. In high school, I was not even aware that International Paper was in Memphis, so that was two dreams in one that I accomplished. Yet, I had a slight hiccup.

The Scarlet Letter P

I remember the day I called my mom to tell her I was pregnant. Even though I owned a home and made my own money, I was terrified to call and give my mom the news that I was pregnant. However, I knew it was inevitable that she would find out. I had to overcome my fear to make the call. Or as some would say, "Put on my big girl underwear and woman up!" After all, I'm an adult, making my own money, in my own house, and driving my car. I'm a woman! I can have a child if I choose to. I'm not afraid to tell her. That all sounded good in my head, but in reality, that pep talk to myself had no impact on me. I was still scared to make that dreaded phone call to my mother. I felt like I was facing doomsday, and I was about to have the walk of shame. Although I did not have the Scarlet letter "A" on my forehead for adultery, I felt as though I had an invisible letter "P" on my forehead, causing the entire world to know that I was unmarried and pregnant, which I felt would result in my mother feeling shame. I knew this was not true, but that's how I felt.

I paced back and forth around the house, rehearsing how I would break the news to her. Looking at myself in the bathroom mirror, I jumped around back and forth, in and out, as though I was doing the pendulum step in a boxing match, trying to shake away the fear. Suddenly, I started sweating. *Was this sweat from my boxing moves, or was it from fear?* I let the toilet seat down and sat on top of it to rest as my heart began to beat faster and faster. I grabbed my phone and typed in my mother's name from my contact list to pull up her phone number. All I had to do was hit the call button, but I couldn't do it. I jumped back up and started my boxing match again in the mirror, sweat beading down my face. I could hear my heart beating as though it was sitting outside of my chest. It sounded like a drum from the MSU marching band.

"Boom."

"Boom."

"Boom."

"Boom."

"Boom."

"Boom."

I sat down again and finally pushed the call button. I whispered, "Please don't answer," but of course, she answered the call. Usually, I would ask how she was doing and how everyone was back in my hometown. Not this time. No small talk. I had to get it over with before I changed my mind. As I sat on the toilet seat, sweating, I started sniffing and crying. I tried to speak, but I couldn't.

My mother asked me, "What's wrong, baby?" Oh my goodness, why did she have to call me baby? Now, I was even more afraid to tell her.

I took a deep breath, swallowed, and blurted out, "I'm pregnant!" I expected her to say something immediately, but there was complete silence. I felt like I was in a library, absolutely no talking or movement from anyone, including myself. It seemed like thirty minutes had passed, which I'm sure was only seconds. Finally, she responded.

"Are you sure?" I affirmed that I was sure. There was more silence for what seemed like hours this time. Finally, she said those words that gave me relief. "Baby, well, you are an adult, and you are working, so I'm proud of you. I'll be here for you." I felt as though I had won the lottery and was filled with excitement and joy from those words. In all the years of my life, I had never been as terrified of my mother as I was right then, a twenty-five-year-old adult. It wasn't that I was afraid of her, but instead I was scared of disappointing her. I thought that being pregnant would hurt her, and that scared me to think of how it would affect her. I was so wrong and had been worried for nothing. And so, my pregnancy journey began.

Becoming a Mother

Being pregnant was amazing! Of course, I was scared and wanted to do everything right as a first-time mother; somehow, it came naturally to me, which may have been due to my experience as an older sister and helping with my younger sister. My first bundle of joy arrived on February 19, 2004. It was the best feeling in the world, and yes, my mother was there! I enjoyed being a mother, especially bonding with my son through nursing.

Throughout the pregnancy, I ensured I ate enough to keep my baby healthy. I did not experience the typical pregnancy cravings that some mothers have. But every single Friday, we would go to Ryan's restaurant for Fish Fridays and the buffet. I know I received enough daily calories, especially on Fridays. I gave no thought to weight gain because I wanted my baby to be healthy.

Once he was born, I was told that I needed to double my calories for both me and my baby since I was nursing. I had no problems with this information, but in hindsight, I wondered if it was accurate. Nevertheless, I ensured that I ate enough to be successful in nursing. As my son grew closer to eleven months old, I started weaning him from nursing so that he could stop by the time he was a year old. I knew nursing was the best form of nutrients for my son, but it was a lot of work, having to either nurse or pump milk every two to three hours. I pumped at home, at work, and when going out with friends. I was determined to have nothing but the best for my son, so I persevered through it, with the plan to stop when he turned one year old.

At that time, I began to think about the weight I had gained. Not only was my son a large baby at birth, weighing almost nine pounds, but I had also gained about thirty pounds from the pregnancy and during nursing. Initially, it did not concern me because just as I knew what my plans were when I was in high school, I knew I would have another child and wanted them to be no more than three to four years apart so that they could grow up together, unlike my siblings and me. Due to the six- to eight-year age gap between us, we did not grow up playing together. Just as I had predicted, my second son was born four years later, on July 19, 2008, and again, my mother was there. As with my first pregnancy, I consumed enough calories during this pregnancy, and I also nursed him for a year, which doubled my calorie intake during that time. My second son was also a large baby, weighing almost ten pounds. As I weaned him, my focus turned toward my weight gain.

The Gym Rat

It's normal for women to gain weight during pregnancy; however, the amount of weight gained is influenced by factors such as food intake, exercise, and genetics. I was getting in my fair share of food. Yet, I wasn't exercising because I was only told to focus on getting calories. As a matter of fact, I hadn't thought about exercising at all during pregnancy or the first year of both of my boys' lives. With my mind reset to having that snatched body, I immediately started working out at the gym to lose the extra pounds I had gained.

I was in the gym faithfully every day. I was no longer "Splinter the Rat," but I was a gym rat. Over the course of ten years, I worked out, hired a trainer, and then hired another trainer after not seeing results from the first one. My trainers trained me extensively, incorporating exercises like flipping eighteen-wheeler tires and burpees, among others. At the same time, I tried multiple diets, pills, and fasting, yet nothing was working. I was so frustrated with not seeing the results that I wanted. I was losing weight, but not in my stomach area, which is where I was the most unhappy and wanted to lose weight. Then, one of my ex-boyfriends contacted me after seeing a picture of me on social media and said, "Trell, you are getting flat back there, aren't you?" By that, he meant my butt. Initially, I brushed off his comment, thinking he was trying to rekindle our relationship. Honestly, I noticed that my clothes were becoming loose, and I was thrilled to be able to fit into my pre-pregnancy clothes again. However, I wasn't entirely satisfied because my stomach area remained the same. It was not until later that it dawned on me that I was now fitting into older clothes because I was losing my butt.

Once my ex-boyfriend's words resonated, I shuffled through pictures looking at my butt. He was right! I was flat back there; my butt was gone, which is why my clothes fit differently. This was not what I wanted; while I was trying to lose my stomach, I lost my butt. At that moment, my workouts came to a screeching halt. It was time to explore other options because losing my butt and having a flat butt was not in my plans. What can I do? I've tried many things that didn't work. Now I just had to figure out what those options were that would have me *snatched to perfection*.

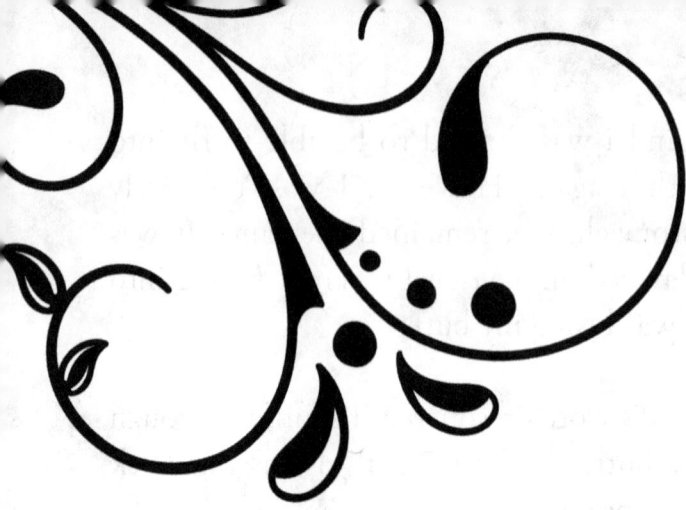

"I began to feel angry toward my doctor and the medical field. Could this issue have been avoided if it had been checked after pregnancy, especially given that I had larger babies?"

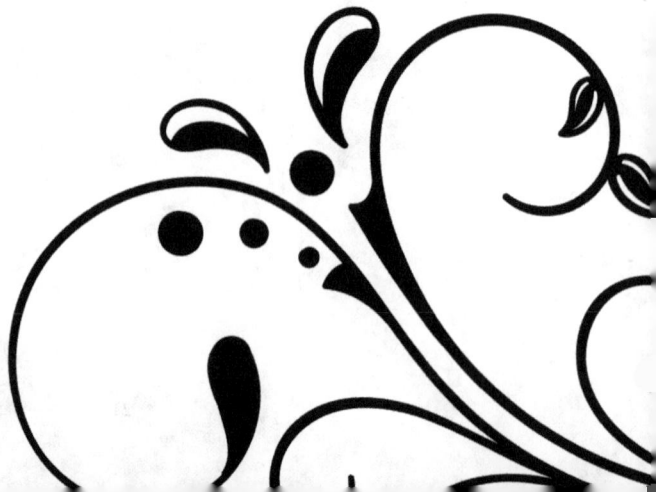

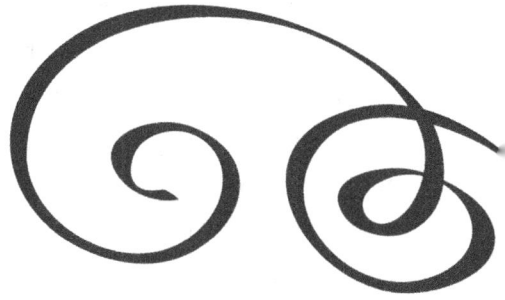

Chapter 3
The Discovery
The Grilled Cheese Sandwich

Initially, I believed I had explored every available option. But I came to realize that I had not looked into surgical options. The reason for this oversight was my fear. I was like a child with a strong aversion to pain. During my kids' pediatrician visits for vaccinations, I was more anxious than they were. Instead of them crying, I found myself in tears for them. I would squeeze my eyes shut so tightly that it felt like they might pop out of their sockets. I gripped a stress ball so hard that it seemed like it could burst. I was genuinely terrified of any pain, and I couldn't stand the sight of blood or anything related to it. So, I wondered, how would I ever muster the courage to undergo surgery? I felt lost and uncertain, but I knew I had to try something different because nothing else had worked thus far.

We Don't Cover It

Although I had medical insurance and was earning more money in Memphis, I was aware that surgery could be so costly.

Despite my fears about undergoing surgery, I decided to call my insurance company to obtain an estimate of what they would cover and to get a general idea of pricing. I also understood that the coverage would depend on the doctor. Still, I wanted at least a rough idea of my benefits. To my surprise, my insurance company informed me that they did not cover the procedure because it was considered cosmetic. They explained that surgeries of this type are typically not covered and can cost $20,000 or more. While I was employed, I couldn't afford that expense.

On one hand, I felt relieved because of my anxiety about surgery. On the other hand, I was disappointed because I found myself back at square one without any answers, which prompted me to research topics such as pain-free weight loss and achieving a toned body without surgery. Unfortunately, most results included diets and exercises that I had already tried, resulting in a multitude of articles that provided little to no help.

Non-invasive

I had been searching for hours, determined to find some information that would help me. Suddenly, buried among the irrelevant search results, I stumbled upon an article about non-invasive surgery options. Non-invasive, in the context of cosmetic procedures, means there's an alternative method that doesn't involve cutting me open with surgical tools. To me, that meant a way to achieve a toned body without traditional surgery. This was precisely what I had been looking for. What a win!

The article focused on CoolSculpting, a procedure that

involves freezing fat. My initial reaction was that it sounded painful. However, I reassured myself that it could not be more painful than surgery. Since it didn't involve blood, the couple of thousand dollars it cost seemed worth it. I immediately began researching CoolSculpting and looked for a location near me that offered the procedure. After finding a clinic, I called to schedule an appointment, and they had availability that same day. I booked it on the spot, hoping to avoid second-guessing my decision.

CoolSculpting

As the minutes passed, my anxiety about the appointment grew, but I managed to stay strong and went to the clinic. Upon arrival, I signed in and was taken to the back for a brief consultation. They asked about my motivation for the procedure, the areas I wanted to target, and what I had tried in the past. The aesthetician explained the CoolSculpting process and what I could expect during and after the procedure. She also discussed the potential side effects and the number of sessions required for optimal results. Honestly, everything she said sounded like Charlie Brown's teacher, because I was focused on one question: Would it make my stomach flat? When she confirmed that it would, I felt a rush of excitement and knew I was ready to begin. I undressed and lay down on the treatment table.

She first wiped my stomach before applying a gel that was slightly cold but not unbearable. Then, she focused on sections of my abdomen and used suction on each area. As she applied the suction, I felt a tingling and cold sensation, much colder than the gel! It wasn't unbearable, but it slowly started to become painful. In my mind, I kept telling myself to endure it because it was better than surgery; after all, I would have a flat abdomen after this! Suddenly, the tingling and coldness intensified, and at that moment, I understood what "freezing the fat" meant. It was so cold that I felt as though I was in a tub of ice, and then my abdomen went completely numb. It was a strange feeling because no anesthesia was involved with CoolSculpting; yet, I couldn't feel my stomach. I was unsure whether that was a good or bad thing, but I was so focused on having a flat stomach that I didn't care.

After the procedure, she performed a massage on the treated areas, which I thought would feel good and alleviate the numbness. The thought of a massage thrilled me, as I desperately needed the relaxation after the procedure; I was more than ready for it. Until I wasn't! The massage was anything but relaxing; it was excruciating. I don't know if it was due to the numbness, the freezing, or both, but I was in excruciating pain for twenty minutes. With every impression on my body, I jerked and jumped. I couldn't wait to leave and vowed never to return. Just then, she showed me the before-and-after results, and I was amazed! I noticed a difference, not quite the flat stomach I wanted, but she did tell me I would need a few sessions to achieve the best results. She also provided me with post-procedure care instructions and scheduled a follow-up appointment to monitor my progress. I smiled, completely forgetting the painful experience I had just gone through, and booked my next session. It took me some time to regain my mobility, but I eventually managed to get up and get dressed.

Later that night, I began experiencing extreme tingling and itching, and the numbness persisted. I thought it might go away by the next day, but it didn't. The following morning, I contacted the office and was informed that what I was experiencing was normal; they assured me it would subside in a few days. However, those few days were the most torturous I had ever experienced in my life. At that point, I realized I could not return, as the minimal results were not worth the side effects. Thankfully, I was able to obtain a partial refund. They tried to persuade me to use the remaining balance on other services, which I refused. I never wanted to return to that place for anything. In the end, I took my partial refund and never went back.

Laser Lipo or Lipo Injections?

I was on the hunt again to achieve my snatched body without surgery. In my research, I discovered other options, such as laser liposuction and lipo injections. The goal was to find something within my budget that did not involve blood or surgery. As I delved deeper into the details on laser lipo and lipo injections, I became intrigued by the success stories and positive reviews. *Why not give it a try? It couldn't be worse than CoolSculpting, right?* I found a clinic that offered both procedures, which was fantastic. They could explain the pros and cons of each option or even suggest trying both! Did I call? Yes, of course! I scheduled an appointment for the next day.

Upon arriving at the appointment, I underwent another consultation during which we reviewed my areas of concern and discussed the procedures. Ultimately, I needed to decide which one I wanted to undergo. Both options were significantly cheaper than CoolSculpting. After our discussion, I opted for laser lipo because it targeted smaller areas of stubborn fat, required less recovery time, and seemed to be less painful. Given my fear of needles, I knew that laser lipo would be the best choice for me. However, at the last minute, I was asked to sign a waiver form acknowledging the risks of the procedure, which stated that it was considered a minimal surgery involving small incisions and potential side effects. *Wait! Pause! Stop the press!* This was a game-changer for me. I understand that everything comes with side effects that can vary from person to person; however, the mention of "incisions" completely turned me off! I was trying to avoid surgery. Why would I agree to have incisions?

At that point, we revisited the option of lipo injections, despite my fear of needles. I now had to take the lesser of two evils, which was lipo injections. I was desperate to achieve my goal. As I signed the consent form, I noted that it included a list of potential side effects. They informed me that several sessions would be necessary for optimal results. I was okay with that, considering the cost was significantly lower than CoolSculpting.

We immediately prepared me for the lipo injections, and I felt a mix of excitement and anxiety, but I was ready for results! The aesthetician took before pictures and prepared the solution while I got comfortable on the table. After cleaning the injection site, she began marking me for the injection. Just like with my children's vaccines, I tightened my eyes and tensed my body in preparation. The injection only took a few seconds, but to me, it felt as if someone had stuck a dinosaur-sized needle through my body. Then she said the words I wanted to hear: "All done!" We repeated the session the following week, comparing before-and-after progress pictures. There was slight progress, but it seemed temporary, as though my body bounced back to its original state each week. By the third session, she wanted to change the solution. Before administering the new solution, she mentioned that she wanted to check something first because she expected better results by the third visit. Oh gosh, if the fear of needles wasn't enough, her statement frightened me.

She asked me to lie on the table so she could check. I froze and wouldn't move, even though I could hear her calling my name. Her voice faded, and I could hear the infamous voice of Charlie Brown's teacher again, except this time, I was gripped by fear. Suddenly, tears brimmed in my eyes. *Why was I suddenly tearing up? Was there something wrong? Did the solution cause an unexpected reaction? My mind raced with thoughts: I hadn't told my family I was here; what if I couldn't go home? What if I needed surgery because of the injections? Why had I talked myself into this?*

I felt her guiding me toward the table, but my legs felt like a ton of bricks, and I slowly dragged myself onto the surface. She began rubbing her fingers gently across my abdomen, moving inch by inch, and pressed into my stomach. My mind raced with questions, especially since she hadn't said a word while examining me. Oh, my goodness, did she just suck the fat away with the injections? Did she remove an organ? Was this a type of lipo injection massage, similar to CoolSculpting but less painful? I couldn't think logically and desperately needed answers, yet she remained silent.

After a few minutes, she asked if I had heard of diastasis recti. I replied, "No, what is that? Am I dying?" She burst out laughing, which helped to ease my worry because if I were dying, she wouldn't be laughing, *right*? She reassured me that I was not in any danger. Still, she suspected that I had diastasis recti, a condition in which the abdominal muscles separate and do not return to their normal position. I needed to see my OB-GYN (Obstetrician-Gynecologist). I anxiously made my appointment, wondering what this would mean for me. Unfortunately, the appointment was not until the following week, which left my mind racing.

Diastasis Recti

The week passed by incredibly slowly. In the meantime, I researched the term to familiarize myself before my appointment. I learned that diastasis recti is a common condition among pregnant women, characterized by the separation of the left and right abdominal muscles, which causes the belly to stick out. While it can also occur in some men, it is very prevalent in women, affecting about two-thirds of all pregnant women. It can worsen with certain exercises. Learning this, I started joining various social media groups, conducting extensive research, and talking to other women. My encounters revealed how many mothers struggled.

At last, the day of my OB-GYN appointment had arrived, and I felt uncertain about whether to be happy or anxious. This one appointment had the potential to answer all of my questions or possibly raise even more. I felt confident going in since I had been with my OB-GYN since before my pregnancies. She delivered both of my children and continued to remain my doctor post-pregnancy, so she was familiar with me and my body.

After signing in and being taken to an examination room,

she came in. She asked how my children were doing and why I was there since it wasn't time for my annual checkup. I began to explain my concerns about weight gain from the pregnancies, detailing everything I had tried, including various diets, personal trainers, and non-surgical options. This exploration had led me to her for an evaluation of diastasis recti. She confirmed that it sounded like diastasis recti, noting how common it is following pregnancies. Then she asked me to lie down so she could perform a proper examination. She proceeded to do the same evaluation that was done with the lipo injections, in which she used her thumb and middle finger and moved up and down my abdomen. The difference was that she had me lift my head and shoulders and used her fingertips, followed by me using mine, so that I could feel what she felt.

She placed my fingers just above my belly button and asked if I thought it felt like space or an opening. I wasn't sure what it was supposed to feel like, so I couldn't tell if it was indeed an opening. After all, my stomach had been a problem for me, looking and feeling the same way for decades. She guided my fingers up and down my abdomen, encouraging me to add more fingers until I was using three, then four. I followed her directions, as she informed me that I had a severe case of diastasis recti. The separation was significant, primarily due to the time elapsed since my pregnancies and the size of my babies. She likened my abdominal muscle separation to a grilled cheese sandwich that slowly stretched apart inch by inch over time. This condition caused a pooch or bulge in my stomach, the same bulge I had been trying to get rid of for years. Until then, I had thought it was just baby fat.

As we continued to discuss the situation, she informed me that if I had been aware of it earlier, I could have done certain exercises to address it or used an abdominal support, such as a belly band, and performed specific exercises while avoiding those that might worsen it, like crunches and sit-ups. I believed these exercises would flatten my stomach, but they were actually making the separation worse.

Naturally, I asked her how I could fix it because nothing had worked so far. Her response made my heart drop: "Due to the severity and the length of time, it can only be repaired through cosmetic surgery to repair the abdominal muscles." *Excuse me? Did she just say surgery? That's what I had been trying to avoid for decades, and now I found out it was my only option!*

On one hand, I was relieved to learn that it was not my fault that I hadn't lost the stomach, previously blaming myself for not focusing on my weight after my first pregnancy. On the other hand, did she really say surgery? Why hadn't this been checked during my postpartum exam? If diastasis recti is so common, affecting two-thirds of all pregnancies, why isn't it a routine part of postpartum checks, along with assessing whether the uterus has returned to normal? I began to feel angry toward my doctor and the medical field. Could this issue have been avoided if it had been checked after pregnancy, especially given that I had larger babies?

The Big Question

Now that I knew surgery was the only way to fix it, would I have to settle for being unhappy about my body because surgery wasn't an option for me due to my fear and the cost? Where would I find $20,000 or more for surgery to correct this "grilled cheese sandwich" *issue? I had recently sold my home. Should I use the proceeds for that purpose? I'm always doing for others and rarely for myself, so perhaps I should prioritize my own needs, given that it was the only solution (due to the severity) and that I had been so unhappy for so long.*

Three months passed, and I finally chose myself and my happiness. With the money from the sale of my home, the only thing holding me back was my fear. Ultimately, I didn't overcome the fear. Still, after weighing the options, which were pretty much nonexistent, I decided to move forward toward my dream of being **snatched to perfection**.

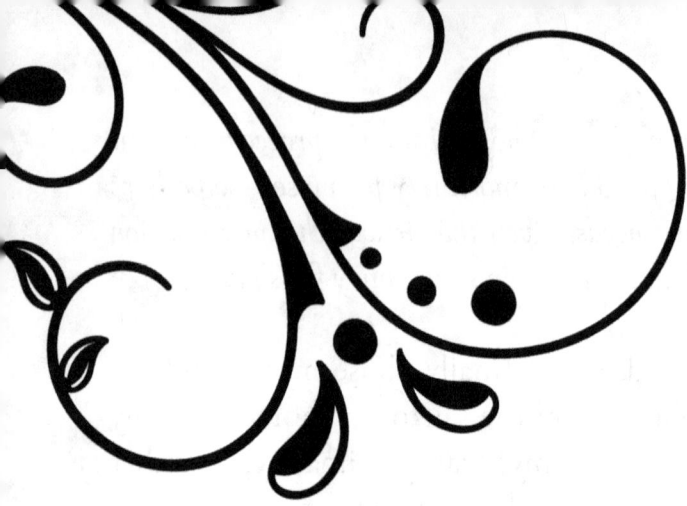

"It's essential to understand that you're not alone... and it's not your fault."

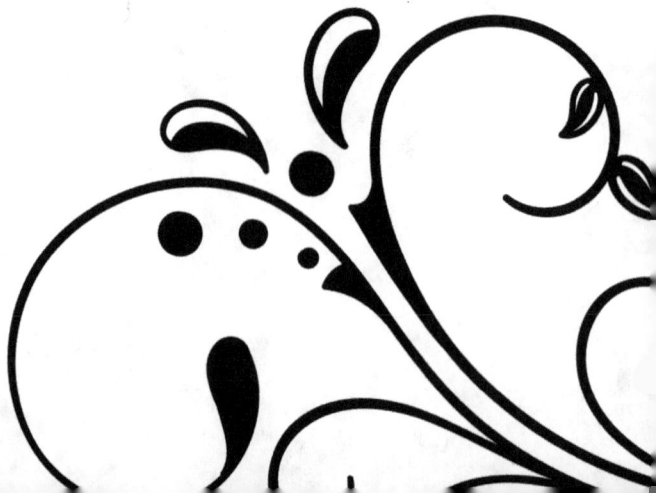

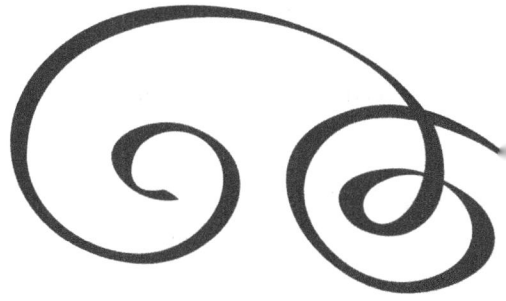

Chapter 4
Understanding Diastasis Recti
The Hidden Separation

Before I ever lay on a surgical table, the pain meds, the rocking chair, and the Boppy pillow rides, something was happening in my body that most people couldn't see, but I could feel every single day. I noticed it in the way my belly protruded, even when I wasn't bloated. I felt it in the weakness of my core, as if it couldn't hold me upright for long periods. I noticed discomfort in my back, which affected my posture and how my clothes fit, or rather, didn't fit. It had a name: diastasis recti.

If you're like me, you might be wondering what diastasis recti is. Diastasis recti is a condition that occurs when the abdominal muscles, specifically the rectus abdominis, separate down the middle. You can think of it like your six-pack muscles being connected by a band of connective tissue. Imagine this band, similar to the melted cheese in a grilled cheese sandwich, being pulled apart under pressure. Unfortunately, it doesn't return to its original form afterward. That's what diastasis recti is!

Diastasis recti can be detected or diagnosed in several ways, but the first step is increasing awareness. Unfortunately, this issue is often overlooked in society, leaving many individuals to suffer without realizing that the condition exists. Once you become aware of diastasis recti, you can begin to address it early and effectively. It's essential to understand that you're not alone; if you're frustrated with your "mommy pooch," there is a reason for it, and it's not your fault. You may wonder how to determine whether you have this condition. There are a couple of methods to assess it, including one that you can do on your own.

Detection

One way to detect diastasis recti is by performing a self-check at home. Although this method is only a preliminary indicator, it can still serve as a helpful starting point. If you have any concerns, please consult a medical professional. To perform a self-check for diastasis recti, "[l]ie flat on your back with your knees bent and your feet flat on the floor. Place one hand behind your head and the other on your abdomen, just above your belly button" (No Tummy Mommy n.d.). Slowly lift your head and shoulders off the floor, similar to doing a crunch. (Keep in mind that this movement may worsen diastasis recti.) As you engage your core, use your fingers to feel the area between your abdominal muscles. If you notice a gap wider than two finger widths, you may be experiencing diastasis recti.

In my case, the separation was wider than all of my fingers, which clearly indicated that no amount of exercise would be sufficient to correct it. After conducting a self-check and consulting with my aesthetician, she recommended that I see my OB-GYN. This is the second, and more accurate, method for detecting diastasis recti: a professional medical evaluation. OB-GYNs and other healthcare providers can utilize their training, along with diagnostic tools such as ultrasounds, to confirm the condition and assess its severity. However, awareness is key! It is the first step to healing, finding answers, and ultimately regaining control of your body.

It is most common in women who have been pregnant with multiples and had multiple pregnancies or larger babies. However, many people may not realize that you don't have to have a baby to experience this condition, although it is more prevalent among those who have been pregnant. Rapid weight gain, intense abdominal straining, or even genetic factors can lead to a similar separation. When the pressure inside the abdomen becomes too high, the central connective tissue known as the linea alba stretches thin. If this stretching goes too far, the muscles can no longer support the abdominal wall as they should.

What many people perceive as just a "mom pooch" or "belly fat" is often something more significant. For me, it wasn't merely about wanting a flatter stomach; I felt a disconnect from my own body. The physical and emotional toll it takes on you is very real. Consistently trying workouts like sit-ups and planks without seeing results can affect you in multiple ways. Many are unaware that, depending on the severity of the condition, no amount of sit-ups or planks can fix it. In fact, doing the wrong exercises can exacerbate the problem. In my case, due to the additional damage caused over the years and the significant separation during my pregnancies, it was beyond repair; a tummy tuck was the only solution.

Beyond the Tummy Tuck

A tummy tuck surgery goes beyond just addressing the skin. Also known as abdominoplasty, this procedure not only removes excess skin and fat but, in some cases, like mine, includes an important step called muscle plication. This step involves stitching the separated abdominal muscles back together, much like sewing a stretched grilled cheese sandwich. This was the key factor in my transformation; my journey was not just about aesthetics, but also about correcting underlying issues. It felt as if a part of me had been reassembled.

Many women are living with undiagnosed diastasis recti, mistakenly believing their bodies didn't "bounce back" or that they've "let themselves go." This issue isn't about willpower; it stems from fundamental changes in the body that require real solutions, not feelings of shame. If we had more open discussions about the medical aspects, physical implications, and their impact on quality of life, perhaps more women would seek the help they need, whether through physical therapy, supportive workouts, or even surgery.

If your belly doesn't look or feel the same, if your core feels weak, your posture has changed, or your confidence is taking a hit, know that you are not alone. You are not lazy, and you are not broken. Your body has endured challenges, and it deserves to be healed. For me, healing meant making the choice to address what had separated, both inside and outside, through surgery. This decision was a step toward regaining strength and wholeness, revealing the woman I knew was still within. That step not only helped me become more confident but also allowed me to feel truly transformed, or **snatched to perfection**.

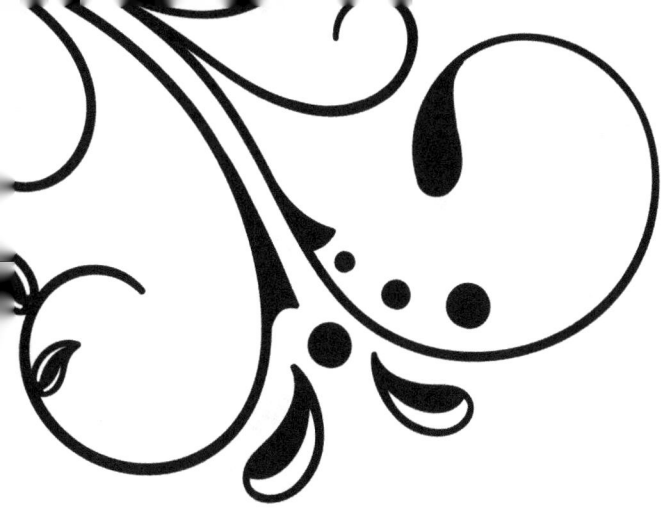

"Sadness and negative thoughts crept into my mind again, but I shook my head to clear my thoughts and fell to my knees to pray."

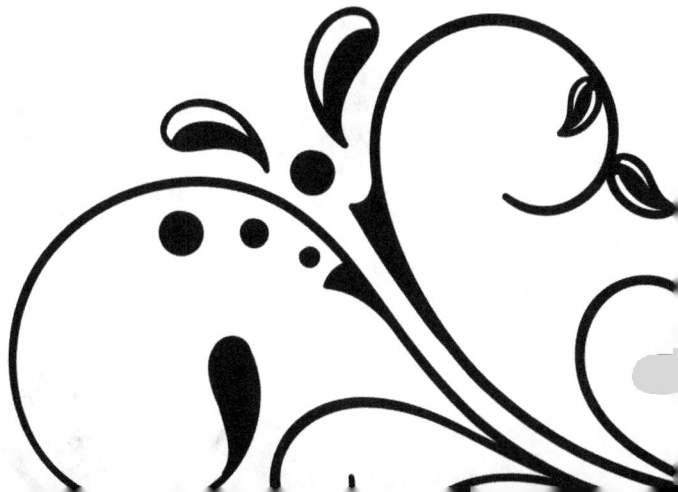

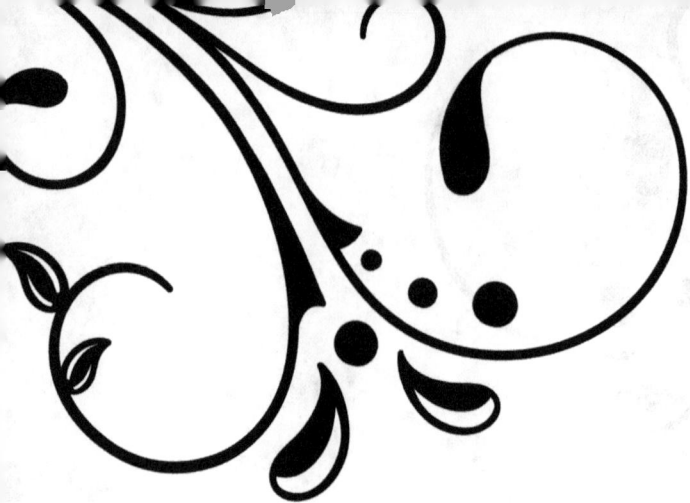

"It felt like I was looking at myself in those photos. The after pictures were stunning, showcasing excellent results."

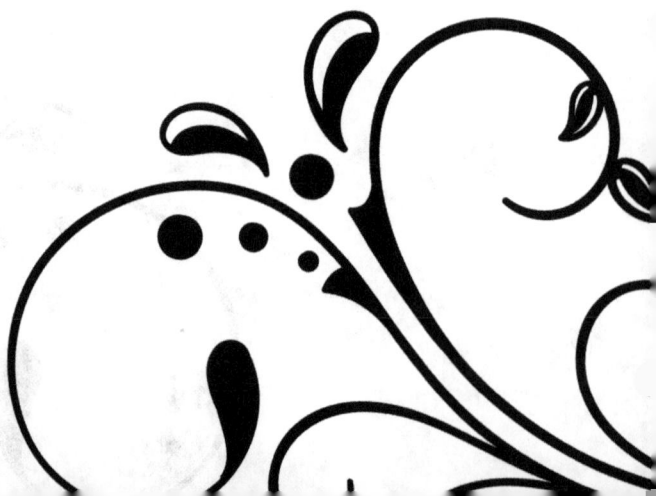

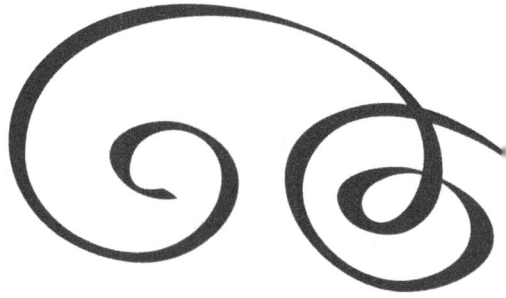

Chapter 5
Pre-Surgery
The Beach Whale

The decision to go through with the surgery had finally been made. I realized that nothing I did would alleviate my concerns about my appearance or the diastasis recti I struggled with. Despite reaching that conclusion, I was still horrified at the thought of undergoing surgery. How could someone who cringes and tenses up at the mere thought of vaccinations possibly endure surgery? Yes, I had given birth to two beautiful baby boys, but that was only thanks to the grace of God and the medical miracle known as anesthesia.

During each labor, I urged the nurses to administer the anesthesia quickly because I wanted to feel no pain whatsoever. However, thinking about receiving anesthesia had me fraught with fear, as it involved a needle being inserted into my spine, which could potentially leave me paralyzed. My fear of needles and pain loomed large, but during labor, I didn't have time to dwell on it. In contrast, deciding to have surgery for my diastasis recti allowed me to take the time to think it through, and I took all the time I needed before I finally made the decision.

Additionally, I needed to find the right doctor to perform the procedure. My OB-GYN confirmed that my diastasis recti was severe and could only be addressed through muscle repair via a tummy tuck. I wanted to find a specialist who understood my medical condition and would not judge me as someone seeking an easy fix. I was looking for a doctor who recognized the seriousness of my situation. It was time to put aside the horror stories I found online and concentrate on researching qualified doctors. I didn't want to revisit Hawaii, feeling ashamed to wear a swimsuit on the beach, as I had a few years prior.

Hawaii

I remember trying on several swimsuits and feeling like a doughnut in each one. I could see the bulge in my stomach, and every part of my body felt three times bigger as I looked in the mirror. Frustrated and angry, I took off each swimsuit one by one. I was really unhappy with how I looked in all of them, whether they were one-piece suits or bikinis. How could I ever go to the beach looking like a whale? I imagined being the laughing stock of Hawaii. At the same time, everyone else comfortably wore their swimsuits, but I would be covered up as if it were winter.

In my mind, I envisioned myself after the surgery in Hawaii. This time, I would be running across the beach like the *Baywatch* beauties in a bikini, hair blowing in the wind, feeling like the only one who looked amazing in my swimsuit. At the same time, everyone else appeared as beach whales. I knew I had to find the perfect doctor to make that vision a reality. And when I finally found the right doctor, it was like a weight had been lifted off my shoulders. I felt secure and confident in my decision, knowing that I was in good hands.

The Search

I searched for doctors who perform tummy tucks, also known medically as abdominoplasty. With so many options available, it felt overwhelming. Having hundreds of doctors to choose from, I realized I needed to narrow down my choices by deciding where I wanted to have the surgery. Through my research on Google, I found that many people traveled to Miami or Mexico for cheaper procedures. However, I also came across numerous horror stories related to those locations. That was a definite no for me! I wanted to choose a local doctor because, in the unfortunate event that something went wrong, I needed someone who could be readily available and accessible. I didn't want to deal with the pain and inconvenience of making emergency trips to Miami or Mexico if complications arose.

By deciding to look for a local surgeon, I reduced my search from hundreds of options to fewer than fifty doctors. While that was still a considerable number, I began the process of weeding through them. I joined social media groups, asked for recommendations, checked medical and Google reviews, and much more. I was determined to find the perfect doctor, regardless of cost, and I hope my determination and perseverance in this process will inspire others facing similar decisions to keep pushing forward in their search for the best care.

Although the price was a factor, my life and well-being were my top priorities. For me, it was essential to find someone local who would be available after the surgery, rather than just seeking a cheaper option. This decision serves as a reminder to myself and others that our health and well-being should always be our top priority, even if it means investing more in our care and attention. Through my research, I narrowed my options down to five doctors with whom I felt comfortable proceeding. I began calling them one by one to discuss my concerns and learn about their processes. Each doctor required a consultation, with fees starting at $100 or more. Only three of the doctors applied the consultation fee to the surgery costs, while the other two did not. This meant that if I didn't choose them after the consultations, I would lose the consultation fees. As someone who works in the finance and accounting industry, I dislike wasting money. However, in this situation, I wanted to make an informed decision and ensure I selected the best surgeon. I knew that visiting all of them would cost me several hundred dollars, but it was important to me.

The first location I visited left much to be desired. I was unimpressed with both the exterior and interior of the facility. While I understand that aesthetics may not be a top priority, the level of care provided might be reflected in the cleanliness and organization of the facility. I needed to see a sparkling location to feel confident about the cleanliness of the surgical equipment and supplies. Whether this perspective was valid or not, it was my way of assessing the situation.

As expected, this location offered the lowest surgery price among the five, which was crucial since my insurance would not cover the costs. Nevertheless, price was not my top criterion for selecting the best surgeon. The second location I visited had a better appearance but lacked friendly staff. I expressed my fears, history, concerns, and medical diagnosis to them, but they treated me as just another patient in their busy schedule. They assured me that the entire process would take around an hour, which seemed inaccurate when considering the pre-surgery preparations, the surgery itself, and recovery time. I didn't want my surgery to feel rushed.

Feeling disheartened, I began to question whether I should reconsider having the surgery at all. But I quickly shook my head to dispel those thoughts. I had come this far: making the decision to have the surgery, conducting thorough research, and attending consultations. I whispered a prayer, asking God to guide my steps and let His will be done. If it was meant to happen, I trusted I would find the right doctor. After all, I still had three more consultations to go. Even though I had already spent $200 on consultations, I chose to remain open to divine guidance for the remaining three visits.

The third and fourth appointments were on the same day. I first visited the third location and was impressed by its size; it felt like a major hospital in its own right. They had multiple wings dedicated to different aspects of the process, including a consultation wing, an anesthesia wing, a surgery wing, and a recovery wing. Doctors were moving swiftly through the hallways, clad in gloves and masks, and I watched in amazement, feeling like an extra in a scene from "Grey's Anatomy."

After checking in, I was called back to the consultation wing. As I shared my story with the doctor, he smiled the entire time, nodding and shaking his head in understanding. He seemed genuinely concerned about my needs, and so far, everything was going well. We discussed the process, costs, and next steps. While I didn't have any negative thoughts about this location, nothing particularly stood out that would make it my choice.

Next, I proceeded to the fourth location. Although it was not as large, it was still a nice, clean, and organized space. I checked in and met with a representative, but not with the actual surgeon who would perform the operation. This was my first red flag, but I decided to give them a chance since I had seen many commercials about this location, and they were well-known with multiple offices across the United States.

The person I spoke to had undergone the surgery herself, so she shared her experiences about the surgeon. She showed me her before-and-after pictures, along with a photo of the fat that had been removed, which was quite shocking to see. I couldn't help but wonder why she didn't appear smaller after having such a substantial amount of fat taken out. It seemed she could read my thoughts or see my surprise because she mentioned that while she had lost weight initially, she eventually gained it back. She had assumed the weight would stay off after the surgery, which raised my second red flag. How could someone who had undergone this procedure not know that weight gain was possible? Did they not inform patients about this?

Another point that caught my attention was her explanation of their surgical approach. She mentioned that they didn't use drains after surgery, which patients appreciated since it meant they wouldn't have to deal with the daily management of drains or their removal. Although their costs were higher, they offered promotions to reduce the price.

They were among the few places that applied the consultation fee towards the surgery cost. With the promotions and the consultation fee applied, the surgery would end up costing about $500 less. I had one more location to visit before I could make an informed decision.

My last appointment for a consultation was scheduled for the next day. That night, after my third and fourth consultations, I reviewed everything I had received and heard so far, as this would be my final meeting. Based on the four places I had visited, the third and fourth options were possible. Yet, still, I wasn't entirely confident in either of them being the right choice for my surgeon. I knew I had one last chance to make the right decision.

Sadness and negative thoughts crept into my mind again, but I shook my head to clear my thoughts and fell to my knees to pray. I asked God to make this last location the best one and to help confirm my decision. I prayed for nearly twenty minutes, feeling the devil trying to sway me and make me question my choice. Deep down, I believed that God had guided me this far and wanted me to be happy, and that this surgery could lead to my satisfaction. I resolved to pray even harder to resist doubt.

The next day arrived, and I made my way to the last location. Upon entering, I wasn't as impressed as I had been at some of the previous sites; this one was located in an office building with multiple businesses leasing suite spaces. It didn't compare to the earlier consultations that felt more like hospital settings. However, since this was my final option and I wasn't entirely sold on the other four, I decided to give them a chance.

To my surprise, the staff was incredibly friendly and professional throughout my visit, from check-in to checkout, and was nicer than the staff at any of the other locations I had encountered. When I was called back for the consultation, the examination room was spotless, and the equipment gleamed. I could practically smell the cleanliness as I walked in.

As I sat down and began to describe my situation, I immediately felt at ease with the doctor. He reminded me of Bill Cosby's character from "The Cosby Show," who had a knack for making patients feel at ease. He greeted me with a friendly, "Hey, Mrs. America! Oh, I'm sorry, Mrs. USA!" This brought a smile to my face, and all my nervousness and tension melted away. He asked, "Now, why does the Queen of the USA need to see little old me?" I felt as if I had known him for years. He seemed to understand my concerns even before I detailed them. "I treat my clients like family," he stated, explaining that he provides his cell number to them and would never perform a procedure on anyone that he wouldn't subject himself or his family to. He then showed me before-and-after photos of patients with similar medical issues and body shapes to mine. Their faces were not visible, but I could see how their stomachs looked just like mine did! The previous location had shown me pictures that didn't feature people with my shape and issues; they were clothed, so I couldn't see their stomachs clearly. It felt like I was looking at myself in those photos. The after pictures were stunning, showcasing excellent results. Some patients even had additional procedures done simultaneously, which gave me hope and confidence.

He examined my stomach and detailed every inch of what he would cut, remove, and adjust. He explained that my belly button would be repositioned and moved up. Confused, I asked how that was even possible. He told me that after the umbilical cord is cut at birth, the belly button serves no purpose beyond appearance. I was still grappling with the idea of moving my belly button, but I trusted him completely. It felt like he was crafting an entirely new body for me, and I thought to myself, "Wow, my body needs that much work."

He sensed my apprehension and reassured me, "I know it sounds like a lot, but it's not. I like to be very detailed with my patients so they understand exactly what will be done, every single touch." He then inquired if I planned to have any additional procedures done, like a Brazilian Butt Lift (BBL), mentioning that he could transfer fat from the tummy tuck to my butt simultaneously. He informed me that, by law, he could only remove a specific amount of fat based on my body. Still, any excess fat removed could be used for the BBL if I decided to pursue that route. It would only add about an hour to the surgery, bringing the total time to around five to six hours.

I told him I would think about it. I had lost my butt when I lost weight years ago, but I never lost the weight in my stomach. Now I was contemplating this because I wasn't happy with my butt. I recognized how much effort it had taken for me to reach this point and knew I wouldn't want to undergo surgery again just for a BBL. He assured me that the receptionist could provide the costs for the BBL add-on, allowing me to consider it further.

I was utterly in awe of this doctor. He was thorough and detailed, even providing me with his cell phone number in case I had any questions after my appointment. By the end of our consultation, my fear was entirely gone! If I had to get a vaccine from him, I wouldn't be scared, as I usually am with vaccines, because he made me feel so comfortable. My initial concerns about the facility being a suite in an office building were alleviated. The suite was quite spacious, featuring several operating rooms, a consultation room, a waiting room, and a checkout area. I had no reason not to choose this doctor, and he sealed the deal for me. Though I had lost several hundred dollars on the previous four consultations, that experience helped me make comparisons. After researching the use of drains versus not using them, I ruled out location #4, which did not use drains. I was 100% sold on the last location!

In hindsight, I should have seen him first, but I had purposely saved this doctor for later because he also had reviews for tooth surgery. I had some hesitations about how he performed tummy tucks and tooth surgeries. However, all of the reviews were five out of five, and he had the best medical reviews and background, which is why he made my top five for consultations. I guess it's true what they say about saving the best for last. I needed to make educated decisions about my choice; after all, that surgeon had to help me achieve my dream of being **snatched to perfection**.

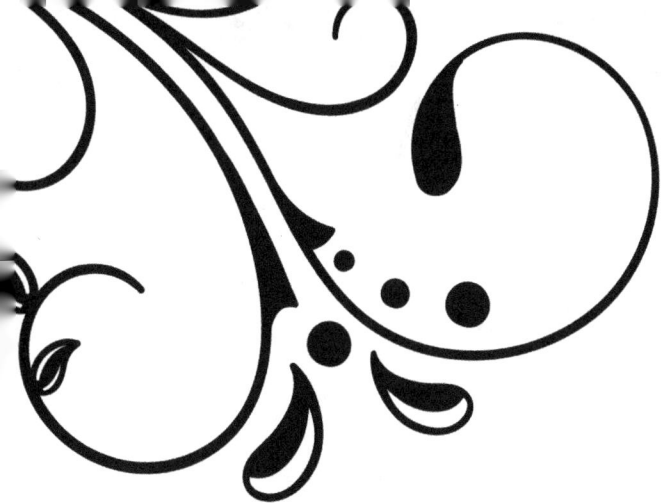

"My determination to overcome these challenges was unwavering. I was moving forward."

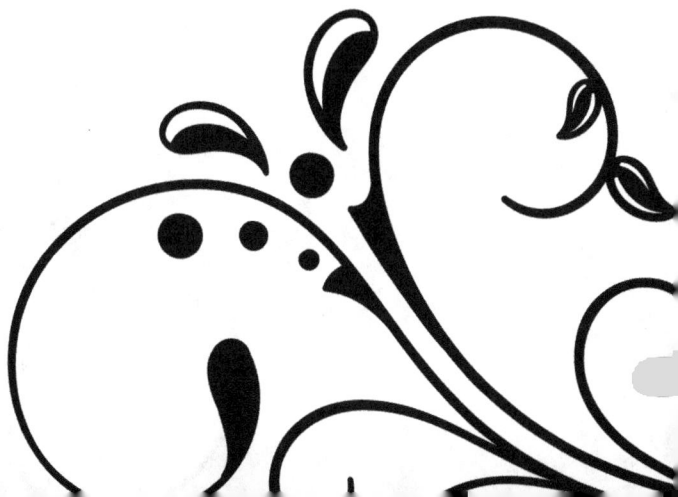

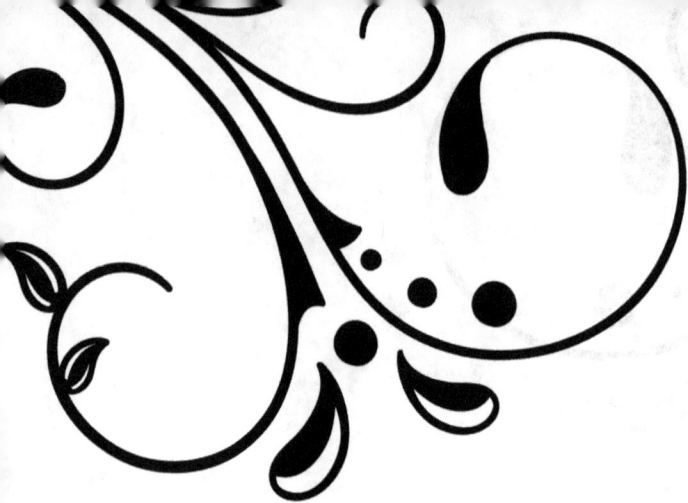

"Oh gosh, it hit me. This was really happening, and my stomach twisted in knots from nervousness all over again."

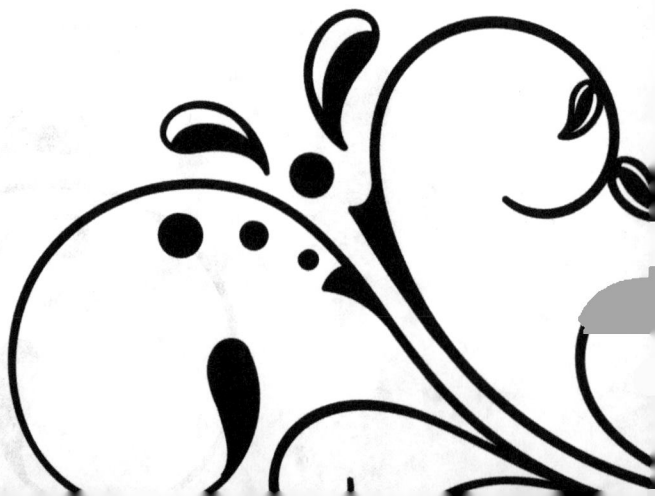

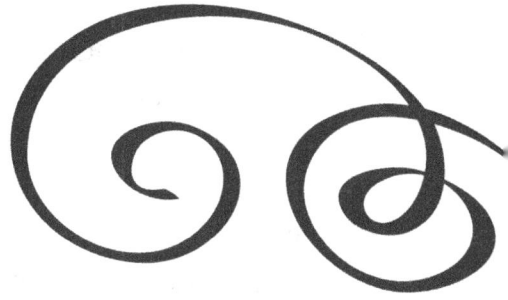

Chapter 6
Decision Day
My Heart Skipped a Beat, Literally

I left the doctor's office after he told me to think about the surgery and call them when I was ready to schedule it. Little did he know, I was already confident, comfortable, and pleased with the consultation, and I didn't need any time to think. As I walked to the receptionist to check out, I booked my surgery date right away!

The receptionist reviewed the pricing, payment options, medical clearance, and the surgery process with me. She also provided the additional price for the BBL add-on, which was $4,000, but I told her I wanted to think about that option. She informed me that I could add it up until the day before the surgery.

When it came time to make the payment of $5,150, with half due upfront, I felt nervous about swiping my card for such a large amount. Despite my nerves, I was ready to take this next step. I squeezed my eyes shut and swiped. The payment secured the doctor, anesthesiologist, and surgical staff, so it was non-refundable. At that moment, I realized there was no turning back or changing my mind after the swipe. However, I was ecstatic to have taken this step toward becoming a happier version of myself!

Declined

Problem #1: My card was declined. Are you kidding me? I had the funds in my account! I had to call the bank to find out what happened. I learned that it was because I had exceeded my daily $5,000 limit, and I needed prior approval for any amount over that limit.

Problem #2: Obtaining prior approval required the signature of the bank's Vice-President, who was out to lunch for another thirty minutes. This day could not possibly get any worse. I was determined not to leave without my appointment, so I sat in my car and waited. When I called back after 30 minutes, the Vice-President was still with a customer. The negativity was creeping in, but I refused to let it take over. I patiently waited for her to call me back, which took another 15 minutes. When she finally did, she approved my transaction. I hurried back upstairs, skipping the elevators, and arrived at the receptionist's desk, out of breath. I wasn't sure why I was rushing so much since they had three hours until closing, but I didn't want to delay my appointment any longer. My determination to overcome these challenges was unwavering. I was moving forward.

This time, I swiped my card with confidence, but I was so quick that I had to do it again. Thankfully, it was approved, and my surgery was officially scheduled. Now, all I had to do was obtain medical clearance and decide whether I wanted the

Brazilian Butt Lift (BBL). I had a physical appointment scheduled for three months later, so I called to reschedule it for the same visit as my medical clearance.

Problem #3: Unfortunately, my doctor was on vacation for the week, so I had to wait until the following week. The receptionist scheduled my surgery two weeks in advance to allow time for medical clearance, which I was grateful for since my primary care physician wouldn't return until the following week. I still had a week for the checkup, so I felt okay about that.

Irregular Heartbeat

During my routine bloodwork (which always makes me cringe since I dislike needles), the technician informed me that it would take a couple of days to get the results, which is standard. I thought I was in the clear until I learned that my EKG showed an irregular heartbeat,

Problem #4: I had never experienced this issue in any of my previous physicals, which I receive yearly. I was perplexed as to why this was happening now. This meant a referral to a cardiologist was necessary. *Perfect timing for another appointment.* Thankfully, my doctor managed to schedule an emergency appointment with the cardiologist for the Wednesday before, explaining that it was required for my medical clearance before the upcoming surgery.

My doctor also mentioned that if I wanted to do anything else for my body, I should consider doing it simultaneously. So, I told her about the BBL. She immediately encouraged me, saying that if I wasn't happy with my butt, I should definitely proceed and have both the tummy tuck and the BBL done at the same time using a fat transfer. This would not only avoid a second surgery but also give me a more natural look by using my own fat instead of silicone implants, which I wanted to avoid. Her support and encouragement gave me the confidence to make this decision.

With this encouragement, I decided to go ahead and add the BBL to my surgery, which would increase my cost by $4,000. Despite my apprehension about undergoing two procedures, I knew I wasn't satisfied with my body, and it made sense to do them simultaneously. After leaving the doctor, I called the surgeon to add the BBL. Was I really about to do this? What was I getting myself into with not one, but two procedures? Yes, I felt terrified, but one thing I always remember my mother saying, and what I learned in church, is that *if God leads you to it, then He will lead you through it, never putting more on you than you can bear.* God knows I have my children, and they need me. So I put my trust in Him even more as I navigated this journey. My faith in God and His plan for me was my anchor in this storm of uncertainty.

Wednesday arrived, and it was the day of my cardiologist appointment. I walked into the office feeling scared and nervous. I had experienced health scares that would warrant a visit to a heart doctor. Questions raced through my mind: *Was my heart about to stop working? Was I going to die? Did I need a heart transplant instead of a tummy tuck?* As I waited in the lobby, I received my bloodwork results from my primary care physician, and thankfully, everything was normal or within the acceptable ranges. This news came at the perfect moment, alleviating some of my anxiety about the EKG results.

Once my name was called and I was taken to the back, the nurse explained what would happen during the appointment. She informed me that I would receive the results that same day unless further testing was required, which eased my mind a bit since I only had two days left in the week. The first task was to get on a treadmill and gradually increase my pace from walking to jogging and finally running so the doctor could assess how my body responded to the changes.

Afterward, I had to undergo another EKG. I questioned the necessity of this second test, especially considering the expenses involved, given that I had just paid over $5,000 the previous week for surgery. The nurse explained that they like to perform their own EKGs to rule out any issues that may have caused an abnormal result during my first test. Although I was initially resistant to the idea of another test and wanted to understand why the first one was abnormal, I was pleasantly surprised when this EKG came back normal!

I felt conflicted about the extra costs (even with insurance); however, I chose to focus on the good news of a normal reading. I now had the paperwork reflecting this result, but I needed to send it to my doctor so she could sign the form, clearing me for surgery. With just one day to spare (it typically took my doctor two days to process the paperwork), I finally received my medical clearance letter, and I could proceed with my surgery the following week. Oh gosh, it hit me. This was really happening, and my stomach twisted in knots from nervousness all over again. In just a few days, I would have the body I could be happy with and would officially be **snatched to perfection**!

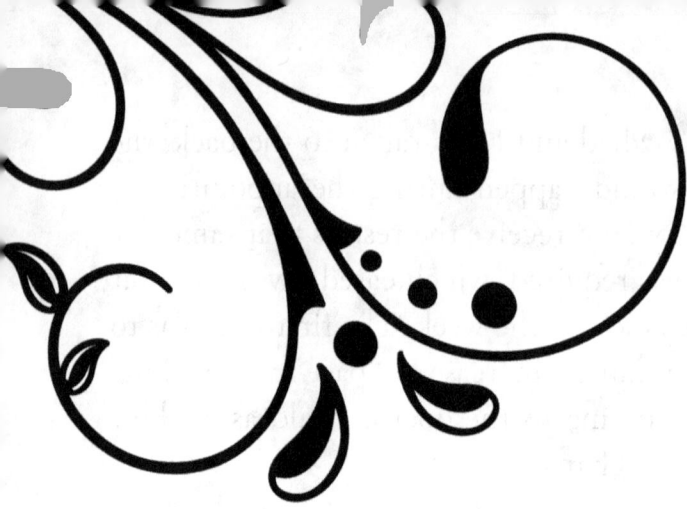

"I told my husband I loved him and asked him to convey my love to my family. After all, anything could happen, but I prayed it would go well. It was time."

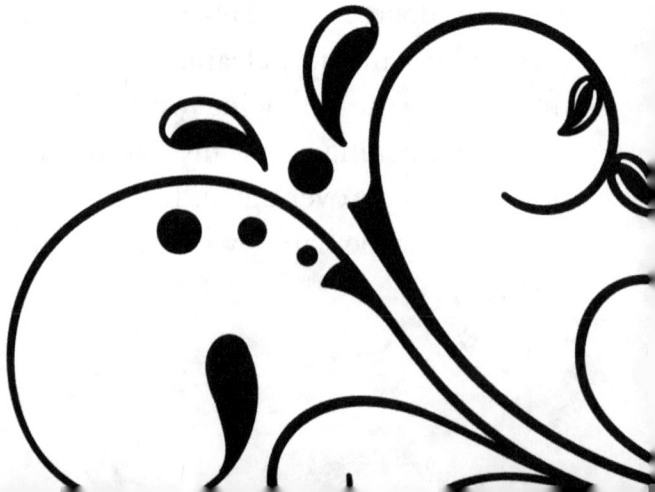

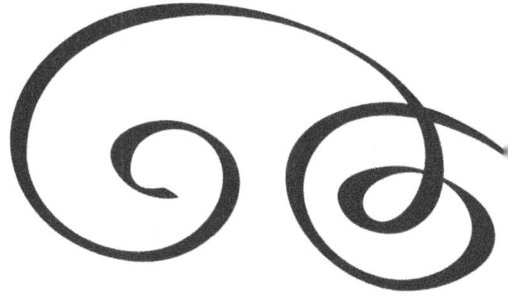

Chapter 7
Surgery Day
Throw the Whole Body Away

The day before my surgery, my surgeon sent me a beautiful floral arrangement, which I hadn't expected. I wondered if this gesture was meant to alleviate any last-minute fears he knew I had or if it was simply a standard protocol. Regardless, I was happy to receive the flowers.

I learned that my post-surgery prescriptions had been called in, seven in total. These included muscle relaxers, a stool softener, nausea medication, antibiotics, pain medication, and more. I was surprised by the number of prescriptions. I dislike taking medicine, so managing that many would be challenging. What struck me the most was the multiple pain medications prescribed. *Why did I need so many?*

Pre-surgery Guidelines

During my pre-operative appointment, I was given instructions on what to do before the surgery, such as dietary guidelines and stopping certain medications and alcohol. I was also advised to shower with Hibiclens, an antibacterial soap.

This was a significant change for me; I was used to my routine and felt out of control following these new instructions. Even though Hibiclens is antibacterial, it didn't feel or look like soap, and it didn't lather. I still felt unclean and wanted to use my usual hygiene products. Still, I followed the guidelines and refrained from using them.

I was instructed to remove any nail polish and artificial nails. What? I had just gotten my nails done a week before discovering that I had to do this! It felt like a waste of money, but it was necessary. Along with these instructions, I received the usual list of potential risks associated with the surgery. I know that there are risks and complications with any surgery. Still, I was not prepared for a two-page document, front and back, outlining every conceivable problem. That realization brought back my fears. *Did I want to go through with this after reading such a daunting list?*

There was no turning back now; I had already paid the $5,000 deposit and the $10,000 balance the day before. The anesthesiologists and other staff had been scheduled, and the money was nonrefundable. I had to go through with it. I didn't even bother reading the two pages of risks because if I had, I might have reconsidered the surgery and wasted the $15,000.

I Couldn't Sleep

It was 9 PM the night before the surgery, and I tried to rest as much as possible to prepare for the next day, since I needed to be there at 6 AM for an 8 AM surgery. However, every time I closed my eyes, I was flooded with images of myself on the surgery table, awake, witnessing the procedure and all the potential complications listed on those two pages. I played calming music, listened to the sound of the beach waves, and watched television, but nothing helped me fall asleep. By 11 PM, I was still wide awake, feeling anxious. My husband tried to comfort me, but it wasn't working. At some point during the night, I finally drifted off, and I remember glancing at the clock; it was 2:10 AM. It seemed like I had just fallen asleep when my alarm went off at 5 AM. I was exhausted and didn't want to get up, but then I remembered what day it was: it was surgery day! Today was the day I would have my tummy tuck, liposuction, muscle repair, and fat transfer to my butt (the BBL), essentially a mommy makeover minus the breast augmentation! I slowly crawled out of bed, still anxious about the surgery and the risks involved.

I said a prayer and reminded myself that by the end of the day, I would be a new person, both physically and mentally. That thought was my motivation to alleviate my anxiety. I envisioned myself dancing in front of the mirror in a crop top, admiring my stomach again, something I hadn't appreciated since high school. I filled my mind with thoughts of how my body would be transformed to perfection in just a few hours. I had conducted extensive research up to this point. Although I felt overwhelmed, I was confident I had made the right decision and was ready for the new me.

The Mommy Makeover

On April 25, 2023, I arrived at the surgeon's office to check in shortly before 6 AM. My husband, who was my driver, also had to fill out a lot of paperwork and understand what to expect for the day. After completing the forms, we were escorted to the back, where we met the surgeon. The reality of the situation hit me again. *This was really happening!*

In the back, the surgeon greeted us, introduced us to the nurse and anesthesiologist, and inquired about my condition. He could see that I was nervous and tried to help me relax with small talk, but it didn't ease my anxiety. He reassured me that I had nothing to worry about and showed me before-and-after pictures to motivate me. He then asked my husband, "You'll stay during the surgery and drive her back, right? She won't be able to drive for two weeks."

Replying, my husband said, "Yes, and I'll make sure she doesn't drive, although that might be a challenge knowing her." They both laughed, which helped lighten the mood.

Next, I was given a gown, socks, and underwear to change into. We took before pictures, and the anesthesiologist asked me some preliminary questions about my health history and explained what to expect during the procedure. I was also informed that I needed to remove my jewelry. That made sense, but I had trouble removing one of the earring backs from my earrings. I had diamond studs with screw-on backs, and one of the backs had come off weeks prior, so I replaced it with a regular push-on back. I didn't realize at that time that a regular push-on back wouldn't work on screw-on earring posts. I found myself unable to remove the stubborn earring back. The surgeon came in three times to check if we were ready, but my husband and I spent twenty minutes trying to get the earring back off to no avail. Finally, the surgeon asked if he could cut it off. I almost choked and shouted, "NO!" He wasn't aware of how much those earrings cost my husband. In the end, the only option left was for him to put tape over my earlobe, which looked ridiculous, but I preferred that over cutting the earring off. So, I chose the latter option and dealt with the silly look.

Once we were officially ready, the nurse took my vital signs and noted that my heartbeat and blood pressure were high. I explained that my levels were elevated because I was terrified. They checked their system to confirm that I had medical clearance from the prior EKG and decided to try retaking my vitals in about ten minutes. At that point, the surgeon asked me to stand so he could begin marking my body for the procedure. It didn't take him long to make the markings, but it felt like every inch of my stomach and butt had been marked all the way around. Looking at the markings made me feel as if I was really out of shape and needed a completely new body. He must have sensed my thoughts, as he reassured me that it may seem like a lot, but it really wasn't. I tried to smile, but I couldn't. I joked that we might as well just throw the whole body away. He laughed, but I was serious.

When the nurse retook my vitals while we were relaxed and laughing, everything was in the normal range this time. Then the surgeon asked a question I was not ready for: "Are you ready?" Of course, I wanted to say I was ready, but deep down, I felt unprepared. He laughed and then walked me into the room with the anesthesiologist. He asked my husband if his contact number was on the form, as they would keep him updated throughout the surgery. I told my husband I loved him and asked him to convey my love to my family. After all, anything could happen, but I prayed it would go well. It was time.

The nurse began setting up the intravenous drip while she introduced me to the anesthesiologist. He spoke to me from one side of the table, while the nurse stood on the other side. Meanwhile, another man sat at a desk, calling out codes and words that didn't make sense to me. The anesthesiologist and the nurse were talking to me, and the man at the table was also speaking, but I didn't know who to focus on. It felt like a cacophony of loud echoes from everyone talking at once. I found myself staring at the ceiling, not blinking, listening (but not really paying attention) to the chatter around me.

My mind was racing with a thousand thoughts, making it impossible for me to focus on what the medical staff was saying. Eventually, a nurse touched my arm, interrupting my spiral of thoughts. She asked if I was okay because I had been staring into space and not responding to her. I was shivering and felt as though I was lying on a table that resembled a freezer. My body became so numb that the only sensation I experienced was the cold tears streaming down my face and onto the table. *Is this what it feels like when people die and their bodies turn cold? Why was I so cold? Was I dying?* My tears felt icy against my skin, and each drop could have turned into an icicle. The nurse asked what was wrong and why I was crying. However, I struggled to find the words to respond to her. Honestly, I didn't understand why I was crying or how to stop. She noticed how cold I was and covered me with a warm blanket, which helped a little.

The anesthesiologist then informed me that he would ask me a few questions and that, in a moment, I would be unable to respond because the anesthesia would take effect. I thought to myself, "Yeah, right!" He first asked for my name, and I was able to respond. When he asked my age, I hesitated, as I had stopped counting after 21 and continued to celebrate my birthday as if I were still that age. He apparently took my silence as a sign that the anesthesia was kicking in and remarked, "Wow, that was fast!" I replied that I was forever 21 and had to do the math to calculate my age. When I finally worked it out, he laughed, which helped ease my nerves a bit.

He then mentioned that he saw I was Greek (a term used to identify sororities and fraternities), just like him. He told me the name of his fraternity and its location. I even asked if he knew someone from my church who was in the same fraternity. To my surprise, he said yes and referred to him as "my boy." That was the last thing I remember before being wheeled back to the recovery room. I'm not sure how long I was in recovery before they brought me back to the room with my husband, but the surgery lasted almost eight hours. I'm grateful I had no awareness of the extended time, though I know my husband must have been worried since it was supposed to be a five to six-hour surgery. Nonetheless, it was over!

I remember being brought back into the room with my husband. I was told I would have about an hour of recovery time. Everything felt distant and blurry to me. Physically, I was present, but mentally, I was not fully there. I struggled to understand what was happening or what anyone was saying, and I felt completely disoriented. It felt as if I had been hit by a truck; definitely not just a little tap, but a full impact. My midsection felt tightly cinched, as if someone had pulled strings on a corset. As for my backside? It felt completely untouchable, literally. I experienced a tremendous amount of hunger, tiredness, tightness, and soreness in my abdomen.

Rechecking my vitals, the nurse said everything was normal. I remember the surgeon coming in, but I'm not sure what he was saying to my husband. I could make out some words, but they didn't all register with me. I asked the surgeon if I had made it, if I was still alive. He laughed and said, "Yes, you and your new body made it out alive." That was all I needed to hear. While he talked to my husband, I slowly became more alert, although I was still in some pain. I let him know that I was hurting and asked if that was normal. He assured me that it was expected and mentioned that I had been given pain medication that would help. He also told me I had plenty of pain medication with the prescriptions that had previously been called into the pharmacy. I remembered questioning why there were so many prescriptions before, but now, in pain, I was grateful for them. Just then, I suddenly felt nauseous. Out of nowhere, I started gagging and vomited into the emesis bag. *Where did that come from?* It happened again immediately after the first time. Was something wrong? The surgeon explained that it was completely normal, which was why they provided me with the bag for now and would send me home with more bags.

The Hunchback

He began providing my husband and me with postoperative instructions, primarily focusing on my husband since I was still slightly disoriented and sleepy. He explained the compression garment I was wearing, the medication, drains, food intake, bowel movements, and more. *Ah, the compression garment was the reason for the tightness in my stomach.* I was advised not to remove it until my follow-up appointment, where it would be taken off. Unfortunately, I realized I wouldn't see my new body immediately, as I had hoped. I felt strange because I couldn't stand up straight and was hunched over with tubes attached to me.

The surgeon explained that the tubes were drains and provided instructions on how they worked. I was expected to walk around, sleep, and eat with two mini football-shaped bags filled with blood attached to me. This was not going to be easy, especially since I hate the sight of blood, and these bags needed to be emptied every hour or as needed. Gross! Although I didn't fully understand how the drains functioned, I recalled from my research that they were essential to prevent fluid accumulation and infection. One of the doctors I had considered was omitted from my list because that doctor did not use drains. I certainly did not want any infections, so I had to tough it out and deal with the blood and drains.

The surgeon then applied lipo foam and a board around the compression garment, making me feel even more awkward and unable to stand straight, wrapped in all this extra padding. I felt like a slumped-over, 90-year-old version of the "Hunchback of Notre Dame," dressed like a football player! After the remainder of the postoperative instructions were provided, I was told I would have a follow-up appointment in a few days. In the meantime, I was instructed to contact the doctor via his cellphone if I had any questions. He would also reach out to check on me.

Finally, I was ready to get dressed, check out, and go home. I was relieved to hear that I could eat because I hadn't eaten anything since midnight the night before the surgery, and I was starving. The surgeon asked my husband to pull our vehicle around, as he needed to show me how to get into the car and sit comfortably after having the BBL

Put Me in Sideways

We didn't think about the type of vehicle we drove to the surgical center. Being an SUV, it was challenging and painful to climb into. It took about five minutes to get into the car and get as comfortable as possible. I was given a pillow to take with me. Still, I was instructed to get either a pregnancy pillow or a Boppy-style pillow for sitting and sleeping. I was not supposed to sit on my butt for a few weeks so that the fat could settle without damaging the newly injected fat. *Wait, what? How was I going to manage this when I had to work at a desk?* At that moment, I didn't understand how this would work. I knew I would use the pregnancy pillow for sleeping to ensure I didn't roll onto my butt, as I was expected to sleep in a recliner for a couple of weeks. However, I was puzzled. *How could I sleep in a chair or work at a desk?* Later, I researched the Boppy pillow and discovered that it was designed like a doughnut, allowing my butt to fit into the hole while keeping it elevated off the seat. That made a bit more sense.

For now, getting into the vehicle was a challenge; I had to lie on my side, which was uncomfortable. As I lay down, my thoughts returned to my hunger. Feeling as though I hadn't eaten in weeks, we stopped at a restaurant to get something to eat. However, I was so sleepy that I immediately fell asleep once I got into the car and arrived home, so I didn't eat anything. I guess I was more tired than hungry.

I slept for what felt like days, though it was only about six hours. When I woke up, I was ready to eat, but I also felt pain as the pain medication had worn off. I looked down at my stomach and butt, hoping to see my new body, but then I remembered I was still wearing the garment. I began to wonder what I looked like underneath it and smiled, thinking that I finally had a new body. It had been a challenge to get to this point, but I made it! Little did I know, the hard work was just beginning, even though I felt like I'd been *snatched to perfection*!

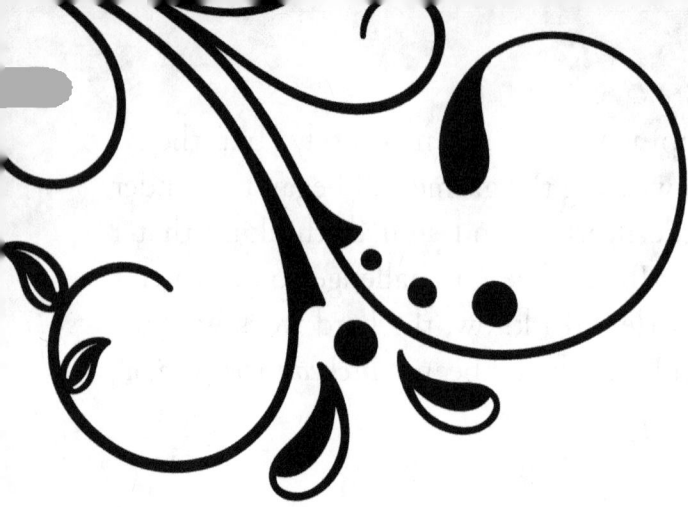

"There had to be an end to this nightmare, but what could help give me some relief?"

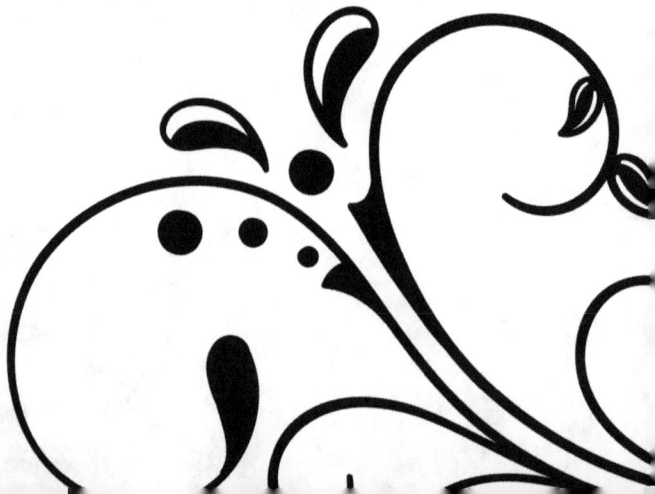

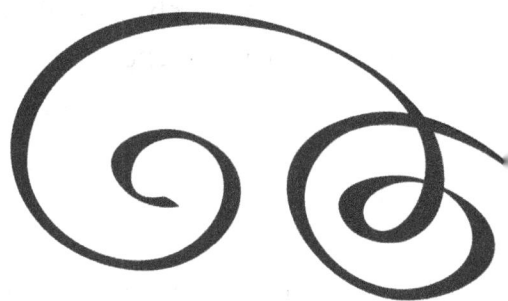

Chapter 8
Post-Surgery
Tucked, Taped, and Totally Over It

The dream had always been to feel comfortable in my own skin, with a tight waist, lifted curves, and a confidence that shines through before I even said a word. However, few people talk about what happens after the surgery. Let me be the first to tell you that beauty comes with a recovery process, and it's not pretty. It's essential to have realistic expectations about this journey, and I'm here to provide you with the necessary information to be prepared.

The First Seventy-Two Hours

The first seventy-two hours after surgery were brutal, worse than I ever imagined. Walking? Not really. I couldn't move without assistance. They gave me a shot to manage the pain, but even with that, the most I could do was shuffle a few steps at a time. It was more comfortable only to sit, sleep, and eat; and if that meant using an adult diaper, so be it. After all, that was part of the deal, right?

Every two to three hours, I had to attempt to walk a little

farther, and each time it felt like I was climbing a mountain without legs, as excruciating pain jolted me. Though hesitant, I had to switch to a stronger pain medication. I saw how easily celebrities became addicted to them. Nevertheless, I was desperate.

Within minutes, the pain medication took effect, and I was able to move. The effect was that I was incredibly drowsy and slept fifteen to twenty hours a day. My husband checked on me frequently, waking me to eat, take my meds, and try to move around to prevent blood clots. After a few days of this, I realized how easy it would be to become dependent on the painkillers, so I decided to wean myself off them.

Weaning

I found myself gradually becoming accustomed to the absence of pain, enjoying more comfortable sleep, and no longer dwelling on anything else. To maintain control, I reduced my medication intake to once a day and fought through the pain when it wore off. I knew that if I didn't control them, those pills would control me.

My husband played a crucial role in my healing process. He kept a notebook detailing every medication I had, the times I took them, when my drains needed to be emptied, the amount collected from each drain, my eating schedule, and more. I was so out of touch with reality that I had no idea all of this was happening for me, and I could never have managed it on my own. My surgeon called daily to check in on my progress, instructing my husband to reach out for anything, big or small.

Did You Go Yet?

I was trying to feel beautiful and whole again while lying in a recliner, swollen and stitched up. During the times I was awake, I struggled to make it to the bathroom. I had to humble myself and wear adult diapers, which was embarrassing, but the pain of standing to use the bathroom was unbearable. I reminded myself that it's all part of the journey, *right?*

To make matters worse, I couldn't have a bowel movement at all, which is an uncomfortable topic that nobody wants to discuss, but it's something everyone needs to hear. After surgery, my body slowed down significantly. I spent days without a bowel movement, and my surgeon made it clear that this could not continue. I needed to go daily or risk further complications.

Each time my surgeon checked on me, the conversation inevitably circled back to the same question: "Have you gone yet?" I kept saying no. They prescribed something to help, but it didn't work. Eventually, my surgeon said I needed to take a prescription shot. Did I mention I hate shots and am terrified of them? But I had to take it to have a bowel movement. The surgeon warned that if I didn't go after the first shot, I would need another later that night. Are you kidding me? Out of sheer desperation, I took one shot but couldn't bring myself to do it again. Then, my husband suggested I try an enema. I wasn't sure what that was, but I thought anything was better than a shot, so I decided to give it a try.

Just like that, in seconds, I was cramping, hunched over, and barely able to walk, but still had to rush to the toilet over and over like it was an Olympic event. I made a desperate dive for the bathroom, forgetting that I couldn't walk that fast. *Should I use an adult diaper?* The thought of sitting in my bowel movements was unfathomable. *Eeew!* I forced myself to get up and move to the bathroom. I moved slowly, feeling like I wouldn't make it, and I barely did. That enema worked super quickly.

Later, I learned it was like a pre-med before my colonoscopy, which I had the following year. What in the world was in this enema that made it work so fast, and why couldn't I stop having bowel movements? It worked too well. I went from zero to full-blown colonoscopy prep chaos in no time. I couldn't stop. I cried, laughed, and groaned all at once. Nobody warns you about how undignified healing can be. I'm sure that's too much information, but hey, don't you want to know what they don't tell you about surgery?

Do I Want My Money Back?

The first month after surgery was challenging. I dealt with swollen ankles, needed to wear compression garments, had post-operative drains, had to take sponge baths, and often questioned why I had ever signed up for this procedure. I was utterly dependent on others for food, support, and help getting out of a chair. I experienced leaking fluid from the drains and adhered to strict no-exercise rules. Yet, it was also a time of transformation. I was learning to be patient with my body and to trust the process, even when I couldn't see any result because, honestly, I didn't see any results at all!

By the end of the first week, it was time to transition from the binder to a faja. I first tried on a size 2X, but it didn't fit. A size 3X was still a no-go; I couldn't even get it past my hips!

Standing there, I felt frustrated, sweaty, and on the verge of tears. Eventually, I had to go up to a size 4X to get it on. How was it possible that, after a tummy tuck with liposuction, I was now wearing sizes twice what I wore before the surgery? My body felt foreign, swollen, and stiff. Still, I kept reminding myself that this was temporary and part of the healing process, at least I hoped it was.

Sleeping was an absolute nightmare. No pun intended. For the first couple of weeks, I literally had to live in a recliner, curled around a body pillow, trying to find some semblance of comfort both day and night. I was propped up like a grandmother, with pillows tucked behind my back, under my thighs, on my sides, and beneath me. After my tummy tuck and BBL, I was unable to stand upright, lie on my stomach, or sit flat on my back. I even took a Boppy-style pillow to my kids' sporting events so I could sit down to avoid sitting flat on my backside. I perched on that U-shaped donut as if it were my throne. The goal was to avoid putting pressure on my newly transferred fat cells, but in reality, I looked like I was dramatically attached to a nursing pillow. Other parents thought I was simply using it for comfort during long games, and I wasn't ready to reveal that I had undergone surgery. However, one parent asked what exercises I had done because my butt looked bigger. I couldn't tell if she was being serious or prying for information, as I couldn't see any change at all this early in the process. This experience wasn't glamorous, but it was necessary for my happiness.

Two weeks after my surgery, my belly button continuously filled with fluid due to its repositioning. I had a Band-Aid on it, but it needed to be changed almost hourly. Eventually, the nurse decided to remove the Band-Aid to allow it to close and heal naturally. I felt nervous, but at that point, I was ready for anything that meant less hardware hanging off my body. Little did I know that my belly button would require more attention later.

By the end of two weeks, I had transitioned from the recliner to my bed, surrounded by pillows to prop me on my sides and keep pressure off my butt. However, this small victory didn't stop my mind from racing. I began to panic about imperfections such as "dog ears," back rolls near my bra, and a new muffin top that had appeared on my right side. "Dog ears" refer to small, triangular flaps of skin that can form on the sides of the waist following a tummy tuck. I had gone from having a pooch to this!

My back bra rolls, fat deposits on my upper back near the bra straps, had been less noticeable before, so why were they so apparent now after liposuction? I had assumed they would be completely gone! Fat hung over my waist. I had previously struggled with a significant pooch due to diastasis recti, but how was that now leading to a muffin top? I was spiraling. Was I ruining my results? Had I wasted my money? When I looked in the mirror, I barely recognized myself. Thankfully, my surgeon had provided us with his number for any questions, so I called to ask why I was experiencing these new issues that hadn't existed before. He reassured me that it would all smooth out in a few months, which relieved me, as I was ready to demand a refund for my $15,000 procedure.

Being in bed by the end of week two, life seemed great until week three arrived, which was pure torture. The itching started. Each day, it intensified, relentless and nonstop. The worst part was that I was still in the faja, which prevented me from scratching as much as I wanted. I hadn't gotten my nails done since before the surgery, so they were in terrible shape. That turned out to be a good thing because I was scratching so hard that I was breaking my nails one by one, digging deep into my skin in search of relief. Eventually, I had to trim my nails completely because I scratched myself until I was bleeding. Yes, it was that bad. I was clawing at my skin through the fabric like a desperate animal that hadn't eaten in days and had finally captured its prey in an attack.

I tried everything to stop the itching: cortisone cream, Benadryl, prescription itch medications, but nothing helped. The only temporary relief I found was from taking hot showers. I ended up taking several showers a day to calm my nerves and soothe my skin. I was in the shower for so long that I sometimes fell asleep. *There had to be an end to this nightmare, but what could help give me some relief?* Then I discovered the pink bottle: a piece of heaven on earth, known as Calamine Lotion.

I had never heard of it before, but let me tell you, it was a game-changer! It looked strange, as it was thick, white, and messy; however, once I felt the immediate relief, I didn't care. It was the only thing that actually worked! I slathered it on like frosting and didn't even flinch at how I looked. I resembled a child who had played in their mom's kitchen, covered in flour from head to toe. But I didn't care because the itching stopped. I could breathe again for hours. When it wore off, I would shower and apply more Calamine lotion!

Lying in my bed... check... no itching... check... Now, life is good! Well, almost. There were still the drains. Each day, I had to empty the drains every few hours, which was cumbersome since they were stitched to my body. I had to be extremely careful not to pull too hard while emptying them, or I risked pulling out stitches. Of course, there were accidents. A few times, I pulled too hard or moved the wrong way, and the pain was intense, lasting what felt like hours. During my week three follow-up, my surgeon seemed happy with my progress. I'm not sure what he saw because I expected to be in perfect shape by now, but I wasn't. Then he informed me that the drains had to come out. Remembering the pain from when I accidentally moved the wrong way, I requested anesthesia, but it was denied. He said, "It'll just be a quick snip, and you don't want anesthesia for something so quick and then have to deal with its aftermath for something so simple." As he prepared to remove the drains, he talked and laughed to keep me distracted while he cut the stitches. At last, he said, "Stitches removed!" I thought, *That was it*. I had been worried for nothing!

My surgeon then asked, "Do you speak any foreign languages?"

I was confused about why he was asking, but replied, "I speak a little Spanish, but not fluently; why do you ask?"

"Because you're about to speak in languages you've never known you could speak," he responded. We both laughed, although I had no idea what was about to happen.

Suddenly, without notice, he ripped one drain out so quickly that I literally heard a loud zipping noise. I screamed like a baby, so loud that I scared myself. I had never screamed like that before. The pain was worse than childbirth; it was worse than the surgery! I was entirely unprepared for that level of agony. I shook and cried, and I probably started speaking in French, German, Chinese, and even tongues, just as he had joked a few moments earlier. Even the receptionist at the front desk rushed in to see what had happened. Anyone in the lobby likely ran out of the building after hearing my scream, probably changing their minds about whatever procedure they were there for.

He asked if I was ready for the second one. "You mean we have to do this again?" I was shocked. He reassured me that it wouldn't be as bad as the first time because I would know what to expect. And then, another loud rip followed by another scream. I don't recall what happened afterward or even leaving the office. I was traumatized and mentally done with it all.

By week six, with the help of foams, a board, and a lot of patience, those trouble spots started to smooth out, including the muffin top that was visible after surgery. However, the mental breakdowns I experienced in between were very real. At six weeks post-surgery, I was cleared to stop wearing the faja, board, and foam. I should have been excited, but honestly, my anxiety was still present. Over a decade ago, I lost a significant amount of weight, resulting in sagging skin. During that time, I lost my butt and still had a stomach pooch. Now that I had a more appealing body than before, I was worried about ruining it by working out too soon. Although I was later cleared to begin light physical activity, I still felt apprehensive about engaging in it.

Leakage

I was in my own bed, free from itching, with my drains removed and trouble spots smoothing out. Life seemed good again, or so I thought. Unexpectedly, I started leaking milk from my breasts, and I wasn't even nursing! Yes, I had nursed both of my children, but that was decades ago, and I had never produced milk since then. So, I found myself back at the OB-GYN.

After conducting some tests, I discovered that my prolactin hormone levels, which are responsible for milk production, were at eighty-four, whereas they should have been under twenty-five. This also explained some of the emotional turmoil I was experiencing, but it didn't provide any comfort since I still didn't know why it was happening. The doctor suggested that it might be related to my lack of a menstrual cycle the prior month, which was most likely due to stress, causing me to have a similar reaction to what occurs during pregnancy and nursing, but she wasn't one hundred percent certain.

Despite undergoing tests, including an MRI to rule out a tumor and extensive blood work, she could not determine the root cause. The only solution was medication to dry up the milk, which left me uncertain about whether it would happen again, especially since I didn't know what had triggered it. When my OB-GYN asked if there had been any recent changes in my life, I honestly replied, "Nothing... oh wait, I had surgery; could that be the cause?" She didn't think so.

With that, I was left feeling even more confused, as the surgery was the only thing different in my routine. Thankfully, once the milk dried up, the issue was no longer present.

However, before it dried up, I experienced some embarrassing moments with wet shirts that made me look as though I was nursing a baby. Milk had seeped through my clothing and dripped down. I felt so embarrassed that I started wearing jackets, even though it was summer!

Let's Try Again

Alright, let's try this again. I was back in my own bed, free of itching, with drains removed, trouble spots smoothing out, and milk dried up. This had to be the end of my struggles. Nope! Despite everything healing and looking better, my belly button wouldn't close. The surgeon indicated that the healing was progressing, albeit at a slower pace than anticipated, and the area was raw and irritated. It turned out to be granulation tissue, and the only solution was cauterization, essentially burning it shut. Just great, another procedure!

Even though it was a minor procedure, I was fed up. I hadn't brought a driver since I wasn't expecting to need a procedure during my follow-up appointment. I didn't want to reschedule, so I went in unprepared, with no anesthesia. I cried before he even started. Flashbacks of drain removal flooded my mind. They gave me something to numb the area (I still don't know what it was due to shock), which wasn't awful; yet, I was already mentally checked out.

Then the nurse brought in the cauterizing tool, which resembled a pen with a needle on the end. When it touched my belly button, I saw smoke and smelled burning. It didn't hurt, but it shook me. The image and the smell lingered in my mind long after I left the office. A couple of days later, when I removed the band-aid and gauze and saw a blackened piece inside my belly button, I panicked, thinking my skin had burned off. It turned out to be just the gauze soaked from the burned belly button mixed with darkened blood, not my actual skin. It even had the unpleasant smell of iodine! It was so traumatizing, but once everything was cleaned up, it looked like new! I no longer saw the internal-like hole in my belly button; it had become just an indentation or inward curve from the ball I previously wore to maintain its shape. I called the surgeon, who reminded me that the belly button serves no purpose after birth. In fact, some people do not have a belly button at all, while others may have a dot or line. Ultimately, it was only for appearance and had no medical purpose. He even shared that it is one way to tell if someone has had a tummy tuck based on their belly button. Now, I find myself constantly looking at others' belly buttons, especially those of reality TV stars, where cosmetic surgery is common.

Finally

At my last follow-up appointment, three months after surgery, I was thrilled to hear that I could finally sleep on my stomach and sides again without pillows. Before the surgery, I always preferred to sleep on my sides. My belly button had fully healed, and I could start taking progress pictures that didn't make me want to cry. However, not everything was perfect. I still had some dog ears on my hips. My surgeon reminded me that this is normal and that many women return to have them clipped. Despite this, I was adamant in my mind that I wasn't going through another surgery, at least not now and maybe not ever.

As we discussed my progress, he took new pictures and compared them to my previous photos. I was genuinely impressed and happy with the results. When he asked if I wanted to schedule a time to have the dog's ears snipped, I hesitated and replied, "I don't know about that because I will never get another surgery." But as I looked at the impressive before-and-after photos, I couldn't help but wonder: *Was I hungry for more procedures, or had I been **snatched to perfection**?*

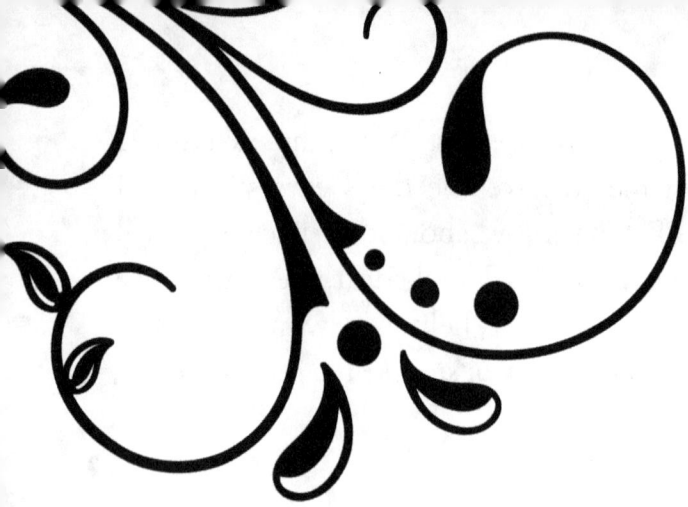

" I struggled with doubts about everything I had been through, and I realized I needed to stop chasing an ideal image and start honoring the efforts I had made."

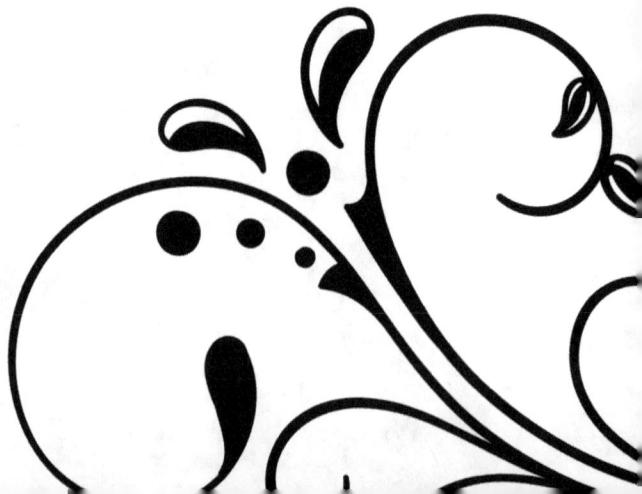

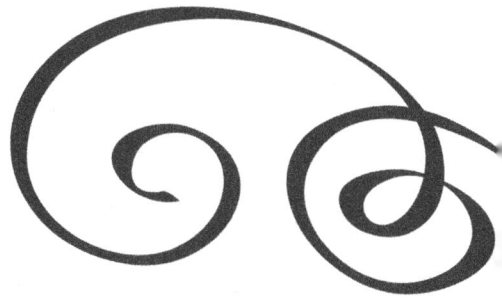

Chapter 9
Acceptance
Wholeness Over Waistlines

Let's have a real talk! This was not a glow-up. It was a grind. I did not get here overnight. Let me say that again: I did not get here overnight! From diapers to drains, bleeding to burning, and an itching that drove me crazy, I faced it all. This book is not about looking cute; it's about educating people about diastasis recti and understanding what it truly takes to get snatched to perfection. Every ounce of my pain was earned for my gain.

When I began this journey, my goal was to regain my body. I wanted to feel confident in my clothes again. I wanted to sit without folding over and take pictures with my kids without having to crop out my belly. I wanted to walk into a room without wondering if everyone noticed "the pooch." I thought that once the surgery was completed, confidence would come rushing in. I imagined I would slip into a dress, take a selfie, and finally feel like the woman who "snapped back," who reclaimed her body and strutted into the world as if she had it all figured out. What no one tells you is that even after you alter your body, your mind might still be stuck in the past.

Shifting My Mind

My reflection changed, but my thoughts hadn't caught up yet, nor had I fully accepted everything. Even after the swelling went down and the compliments started pouring in, I still found myself nitpicking in front of the mirror. *Was my belly button healing properly? Why were the scars still dark? What are these "dog ears" forming on my hips?* There were moments of doubt and times when I was hunched over in pain, questioning whether I had made a mistake. I sat in a recliner wearing an adult diaper, wondering how I ended up there, struggling with itching, crying, panicking over fluid buildup, or fearing that my surgery would be canceled due to an EKG.

Some days felt like I had broken myself instead of fixed myself. However, with every phase, every drain, every scar, every faja, foam board, and hot shower, there was a chapter in my rebirth. I didn't just change my body; I changed my relationship with it. The truth is, I had to unlearn what I thought "snatched" meant. Snatched to perfection wasn't just about how I looked; it was about what I survived.

For so long, perfection was equated with having no flaws, stretch marks, sagging skin, or loose skin. It meant having a tiny waist, smooth curves, and everything looking perfectly lifted. However, even after I underwent a tummy tuck, I still had the scar as a reminder of the surgery. It was located on my waistline, so it wasn't visible even in a bikini. Yet still, I felt the urge to cover it up, perhaps with a tattoo. I struggled with doubts about everything I had been through, and I realized I needed to stop chasing an ideal image and start honoring the efforts I had made.

The first time I looked at my scar without flinching was a moment of acceptance. The first time I walked out without compression garments under my clothes, that was acceptance. The first time I let my husband touch my stomach without tensing up or hiding, it was healing. The first time I realized that my self-image is defined by my perception, not by others, that was a healing moment.

When I finally began to love my body, not because it was perfect, but because it was mine, I experienced true beauty. I came to understand that confidence doesn't depend on waist measurements; it thrives in ownership. It lies in being able to say, "Yes, I went through this. Yes, I chose this path. Yes, my body has endured so much, and I love her for it." For the first time in years, I feel like I am walking in my own skin, not in someone else's vision of who I should be, nor a filtered representation of post-baby bodies or social media ideals. I am just me: strong, empowered, and self-defined.

This book is about liberation from other people's opinions, from my own inner critic, and from the issues that arise with our bodies, such as diastasis recti. It addresses the shame that society places on motherhood, surgery, and the desire for more. My waistline and body may not be flawless, but I am whole. If that isn't what snatched to perfection means, I don't know what does.

If you've journeyed this far with me, I sincerely thank you. Thank you for walking with me through every raw, unfiltered moment, from pain and panic to procedures and healing, and the hard-won confidence that followed. Writing this was not easy; reliving those moments was even harder. But it was necessary. I overcame so much that I didn't realize until I began to write, and my emotions and thoughts spilled out.

I did not write *Snatched to Perfection* to glamorize cosmetic surgery. I wrote it to reveal the truth about what we go through mentally, physically, emotionally, and spiritually when we feel dissatisfied with ourselves. I wanted to educate my readers that there may be underlying reasons for their feelings, such as diastasis recti. I wanted to voice the things that many people only whisper about. I aimed to shine a light on aspects of the process that rarely make it to social media or television, such as the tears, fears, diapers, and scars.

I wrote this for those (male or female) who sit in silence, questioning whether they are the only ones feeling as though their bodies have betrayed them after pregnancy or weight gain. I wrote this for those considering surgery who feel guilty for wanting more. I wrote this for those who've done everything "right" with diet and exercise but still can't close the gap in their core, nor in how they see themselves. You're not alone. You're not crazy. You are not broken. You don't have to apologize for wanting more or explain why you chose the path you did. You don't need to feel ashamed of your scars, stretch marks, or your story. You don't have to conform to anyone else's version of perfect. You are becoming, in your own time and in your own way. That, my dear, is the true definition of **snatched to perfection**.

Whether you choose surgery, therapy, fitness, or simply radical self-love, I want you to remember: your body is not the enemy; it is your vessel, your memory keeper, your battleground, and your home. You deserve to feel powerful in your own skin. Thank you for allowing me to share my truth. Now, give yourself permission to embrace your own.

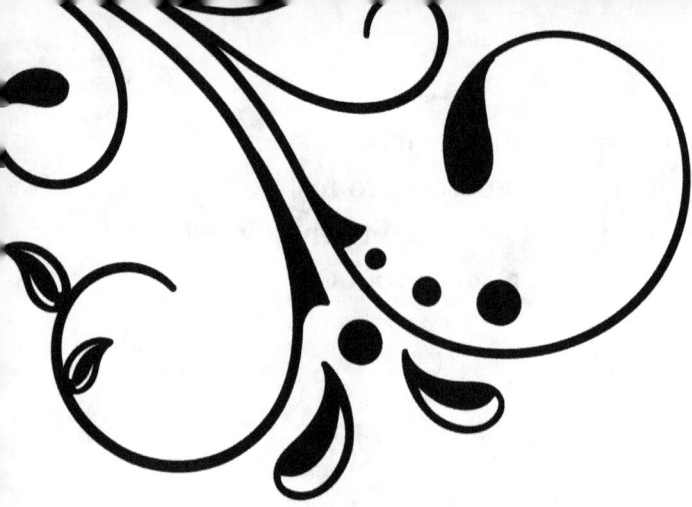

"You're not alone.
You're not broken.
And you don't have to
explain your healing
journey to anyone."

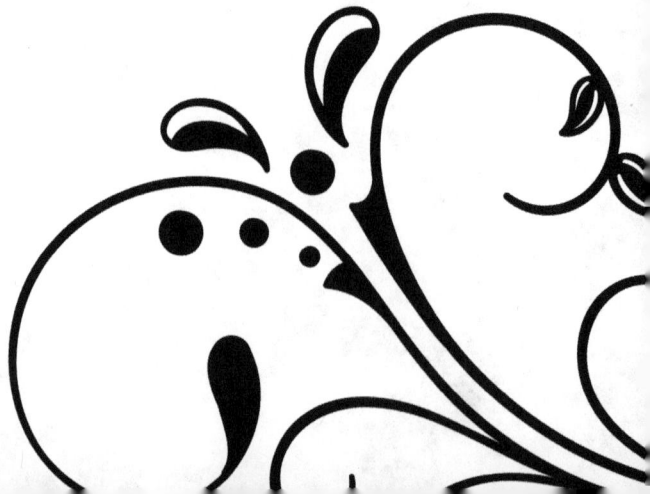

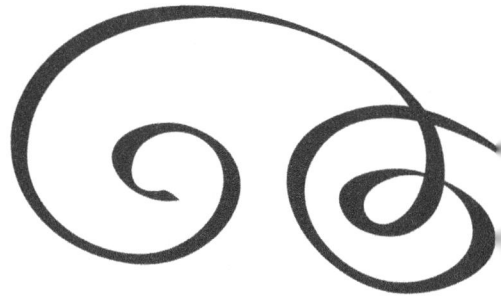

Conclusion
The End and Beginning of Me

This is the end of this story, but it marks the beginning of my new story. My experience started with a condition that many people struggle to pronounce: diastasis recti. This issue was not just about my appearance; it affected my function, caused pain, and created a disconnect between me and my own core. It was a silent separation that left me feeling broken in ways I often couldn't articulate. Like many women, I felt as though I had been handed a postpartum body with no clear roadmap for healing, only unrealistic expectations to "snap back" into shape.

When trainers, diets, exercises, and pills didn't yield the results I hoped for, I became aware of diastasis recti. That realization hit me hard; I understood that this was not something I could fix with willpower alone. It took immense courage to decide to turn to cosmetic surgery. This choice was not made out of vanity but out of necessity. It became my path toward restoration and a challenging journey to feeling whole again.

I faced judgment from others who had no idea what it truly took to reclaim my body. It demanded tough conversations with myself about my worth and confidence as I navigated the dilemma of whether I was chasing society's ideals or genuinely healing from the inside out. I experienced moments of self-doubt and battled with my own self-image. But through it all, I persevered, knowing that this journey was for me.

Many people were unaware of the emotions I experienced while persevering and accomplishing my goals. While I seemed successful, I often felt mentally checked out and incomplete. When we have dreams and aspirations, it's crucial not to let others control our minds or influence our success. Although I struggled with my body image, I pushed through because I had children depending on me. My children were my motivation and my reason for continuing, even when the journey seemed too difficult. Prioritizing them helped me stay on my path to success. Everything I have done in life has been for their sake and guided by God. I kept God in mind at every step, helping me navigate uncertainty, fear, and difficult emotions.

I have grown both emotionally and mentally, which are vital aspects of my development. If you don't accept yourself mentally, your body image won't matter. It's all about mindset. I've also learned that cosmetic surgery isn't a shortcut; it isn't a quick fix that brings self-love. Instead, it amplifies the truth you carry inside. For me, it revealed a woman ready to embrace her story, flaws, scars, and all. I now feel more confident when I look in the mirror, whether I'm clothed or not. What others say about me no longer affects me as it once did because I have evolved. My perception of myself now matters more than how others perceive me. This growth in self-acceptance is a journey that can inspire and give hope to others.

Surgery was not the end; it was just the gateway to achieving my desired body. I still spend several days each week at the gym to maintain my results and tone my body because surgery alone couldn't achieve that. I am no longer the negative label "Splinter the Rat," but rather the positive title "Gym Rat."

Again, this book isn't just about my waistline or the tightness of my core; it's about the softening of my spirit. It reflects the strength it took to admit I needed help and the courage to choose myself repeatedly. No, this is not the end; instead, it is a beginning. It marks the moment I stop trying to "fix" myself and start fully living in the body I fought to reclaim. It's the point where I can say, "The work is done. Now, I enjoy the woman I have become."

Diastasis recti changed how I moved; surgery changed how I looked, and healing transformed everything. Whether you're dealing with diastasis recti, considering surgery, or simply learning to love your reflection again, remember this: You're not alone. You're not broken. And you don't have to explain your healing journey to anyone.

This is the beginning of me: whole, healed, and finally *snatched to perfection*. Remember, the key to this transformation was the journey of self-acceptance. You, too, can discover this self-acceptance and embark on your own journey to feeling whole and healed.

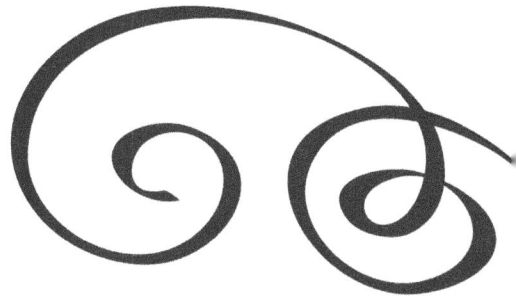

Bonus Survival Guide
Healed, Not Just Snatched

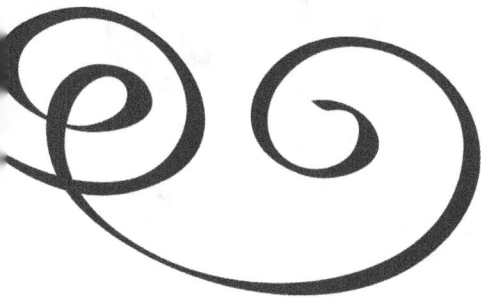

Let's be honest: healing isn't a glamorous process. It goes beyond simply wearing compression garments, fajas, or taking progress pictures. Through the pain medication, sleepless nights, relentless itching, moments of body image struggles, you ask, "Did I make a mistake?" Besides the physical healing, it's a journey that encompasses emotional, mental, and spiritual healing. *However, please note that this guide is not a substitute for professional medical advice. Always consult your healthcare provider for personalized guidance.* That's why I'm sharing a genuine survival guide with you, not the sugar-coated version or what the clinic might tell you, but the honest insights I wish someone had shared with me before going through this journey. As someone who has undergone cosmetic surgery and experienced the ups and downs of recovery, my hope is to help you heal in every way. You will benefit from this guide if:

- You're struggling with your body image.
- You're preparing for surgery and feeling anxious.
- You're already post-op and wondering, "Is this normal?"
- You want to maintain your faith and sanity throughout it all.

From one fighter to another: You've got this! Even when it feels overwhelming, remember that you are not alone. Together, we can survive and heal, so I say we've got this! Together, we share the same struggles and victories.

A Survival Guide for Body, Mind & Spirit

<u>Mindset Reminders</u>
- This season is temporary; it is not your whole story.
- You've survived 100% of your hardest days so far. This one is no different.
- You're not behind; you're rebuilding.
- You don't have to do everything today. Just focus on the next right thing.

Prompt 1: In the following journal pages, take a moment and express your thoughts concerning each phrase.

<u>Empowering Beliefs</u>
- Progress is still progress, even when it's slow.
- It's okay to rest. Healing and strength can happen in stillness, too.
- Feeling overwhelmed doesn't mean you're failing; it means you're human.
- Even in the dark, seeds are growing.

Prompt 2: What are some empowering beliefs that help you when you struggle? How can these empowering belief help champion you toward your goals? Write your thoughts on the following journal pages.

<u>Practical Tips for Handling Challenges</u>

- Acknowledge the hardships.
  - Don't suppress your feelings; feel them, name them, own them.
  - Write them down, say them out loud, or talk to someone.
  - Remind yourself: "What I'm feeling is valid, but it doesn't have to define me."
- Control the controllable.
  - Ask yourself: "What's one small thing I can do right now?"
  - Focus on your routine: eat, hydrate, sleep, and move, even in small doses.
- Set micro-goals.
  - Break tasks down into tiny, manageable steps.
  - Tackle them one by one and notice your progress.
  - Instead of saying, "Fix my life," choose to take a walk, call a friend, or express your feelings through journaling for five minutes.
- Stay connected.
  - Isolation feeds struggle. Reach out, even just to say, "Hey, I need someone to hear me."
  - Join support groups, whether in person or virtually, with others facing similar challenges.
- Limit negativity.
  - Protect your peace: unfollow, mute, or take a break from draining media or people.
  - Replace toxic input with positive influences, such as uplifting podcasts, music, or affirmations.

Prompt 3: Take a moment and plan which steps you want to apply to your life now and how you will do it.

Self-Care & Mindset Practices

- Journal: Dump your thoughts to clear your mind.
- Sunlight & movement: A quick walk can reset your mood.
- Gratitude list: Write down three things going right, no matter how small.
- Read or listen: Choose something that uplifts or inspires you.
- Affirmations: Speak kind truths to yourself daily.
  - "I am allowed to be a work in progress."
  - "I am doing the best I can, and that's enough."

Supporting Someone Else

- Avoid saying the following.
  - "At least..."
  - "It could be worse."
- Instead, say the following.
  - "I'm here for you. No pressure to talk, but I'm listening if you need me."
  - "You don't have to be strong for me. Let's be real."
  - "Is there one thing I can take off your plate?"

Final Motivation:

As this guide comes near to its close, allow me to motivate you with these words.

- You are not weak for struggling; you are strong for continuing.
- One day, this pain will become part of your power.
- Keep going. You're closer than you think.
- Above all: Pray without ceasing!

Prompt 4: We will end with a prayer, but before we do. take a moment to consider the following.

- What self-care and mindset practices will you implement as you face your current challenges.
- What are three things you can add to your gratitude list right now?
- What affirmations make you feel powerful?
- Reflecting on past experiences, how did it feel when someone supported you during a tough time? What did you appreciate most about their support?
- How can you support someone who is currently facing their challenge?
- What are some ways you can show someone that you are there for them without applying pressure to talk?
- How can you identify practical ways to help someone else by taking something off their plate?
- What does it mean to you to acknowledge your struggles as a sign of strength?
- How can you reframe your current pain or challenges into a source of personal power?
- In what ways can you remind yourself to keep pushing forward during difficult times?
- How can you track your progress and reflect on the moments when you feel closer to overcoming your challenges?
- How will you utilize the motivational phrases provided? Will you rewrite them and post them on your bathroom mirror, in your prayer closet, or on your task board? Choose and execute according to your choice.

Write your responses on the following journal pages.

I have chosen to end this book with a prayer and provide you with an opportunity to write your own. Below is my prayer, but in the final journal pages, I invite you to write your own. Whether it is a prayer for peace with where you are, to make the right decisions, or a need for help in the process, write honestly. He is listening. After you have written your prayer, be sure to check out the **About the Author** section at the end to learn more about me.

A Prayer for Confidence, Healing, and Peace with My Body

Dear God,

You see me, all of me. Not just the version I show to the world, but also the parts I hide: the shame, the fear, the frustration, and the exhaustion of never feeling "enough." Lord, I confess that I have battled with my body.

I have hated the mirror. I have allowed the voices of comparison and perfection to steal my peace. I have cried over stretch marks, loose skin, and features that no one else sees as broken but me. I am tired of carrying this burden. I am exhausted from feeling that I have to fix everything to be worthy. Even through the process of cosmetic surgery, the pain, the pressure, and the recovery, I have learned that physical changes do not always heal emotional wounds. So, I bring it all to You: the fear, the insecurity, the questions, the healing, and the scars, both inside and out.

God, help me separate my value from my appearance. Help me understand that changing my body does not change my identity in You. Give me strength on this journey, not just physical strength, but also emotional courage and spiritual grounding. When I feel scared, remind me that I am not alone. When I feel weak, support me. When I start to doubt myself again, whisper the truth to me louder than the lies. Let me walk in confidence, not because I look perfect, but because I know I am loved, whole, and seen by You. Let my healing, inside and out, be a testimony, not of vanity, but of courage, survival, and the choice to take control of my happiness in a world that tells me I cannot. Thank You for loving me, every version of me: past, present, and future.

In Jesus's name, AMEN.

Final Prompt: Release all you feel into your prayer. Write your prayer on the following journal pages.

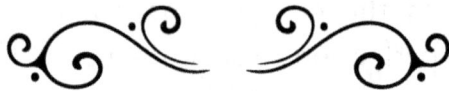

Reminder

Be sure to follow me on all social media channels at Author Trell Taylor (@authortrelltaylor). Join my group as we have honest discussion surrounding body issues, confidence, healing, and peace. Connect with me to join your panels or invite me to speak at your events. You can reach me at AuthorTrellTaylor@gmail.com. I am more than happy to help the next person overcome the challenges I have overcome.

Bibliography

1. n.d. No Tummy Mommy. Accessed November 1, 2025. https://www.luxfit.ca/notummymummy/.
2. n.d. Urban Dictionary. Accessed June 16, 2025. https://www.urbandictionary.com/define.php?term=snatched.

About the Author

Trell Taylor, formerly Yolandria Katrell Taylor, is the CEO and founder of Taylor Made to Travel, LLC, and YoKa Global Realty, LLC, as well as a corporate accountant. She holds bachelor's degrees in Management and General Business Administration from Mississippi State University, as well as a Master of Business Administration in Accounting from the University of Phoenix. Also, she is a member of the illustrious Zeta Phi Beta Sorority, Inc. and very actively involved in numerous associations including the National Black MBA Association and Society for Human Resource Management (SHRM).

Her commitment to help people spans across every aspect of her life and is evident in several notable awards that she has received. As she continues to share her story, she is committed to educating individuals about the realities of the challenges we face and how to overcome them while providing practical solutions. You can connect with the author via email at AuthorTrellTaylor@gmail.com or via social media at Author Trell Taylor (@authortrelltaylor).